Bladder Cancer

A CLEVELAND CLINIC GUIDE

Information for Patients and Caregivers

Derek Raghavan, M.D., Ph.D.
and Kathleen Tuthill

Illustrations by Bill Garriott

Cleveland Clinic Press
Cleveland, Ohio

Bladder Cancer

A CLEVELAND CLINIC GUIDE

Contact:
Cleveland Clinic Press
9500 Euclid Avenue NA32 / Cleveland, Ohio 44195
216-445-5547 / delongk@ccf.org
www.clevelandclinicpress.org

This book is not intended to replace personal medical care and supervision. There is no substitute for the experience and information that your doctor can provide. Rather, it is our hope that this book will provide additional information to help people understand the nature, diagnosis, and treatment of bladder cancer.

Proper medical care always should be tailored to the individual patient. If you read something in this book that seems to conflict with your doctor's instructions, contact your doctor. Since each case is different, there may be good reasons for individual treatment to differ from the information presented in this book. If you have any questions about any treatment in this book, consult your doctor.

The patient names and cases used in this book are composites drawn from several sources.

Library of Congress Cataloging-in-Publication Data

Raghavan, Derek.
Bladder cancer: A Cleveland Clinic guide :
Information for patients and caregivers / Derek Raghavan.
p. cm.

Includes bibliographical references and index.

ISBN 978-1-59624-060-5 (alk. paper)

1. Bladder – Cancer – Popular works. I. Title.

RC280.B5R34 2008   616.99′462 – dc22   2007052211

Cover and book design: J. Michael Myers
Illustrations: Bill Garriott, Cleveland Clinic Center for Medical Art and Photography

Dedication

To my mother, Betty Raghavan, who has faced life
and death with courage and dignity.
– DR

To Beth, whose journey inspired me to care about
bladder cancer, and to my parents, who inspired me
to care about writing.
– KT

And …

To all those with bladder cancer and their loved ones.
May you be blessed with hope and excellent care.
– Derek Raghavan and Kathleen Tuthill

CONTENTS

Acknowledgments

The authors would like to thank Cleveland Clinic
and the Cleveland Clinic Press staff for providing
information, resources, and support. Our thanks go
as well to Jennifer Stonebrook of the Hospice of the
Western Reserve and to Judy Levendula, L.I.S.W.,
and the Hospice team of Cleveland Clinic
for their generous interviews.

Special thanks to Mary Jo Gurin of Cleveland Clinic
for her generous help in getting this
manuscript "to the end."
– KT

Introduction

The bladder is a hollow organ nestled in the lower abdomen that serves as a storage container for urine, the liquid waste produced by the kidneys. The inner tissue of the bladder is surrounded by an outer layer of muscle that tightens to increase the pressure in the bladder when one is about to pass urine, forcing the urine to pass from the bladder into the urethra (the flexible tube that carries urine from the bladder to the point of urination) and out of the body. Cancer that arises in the bladder is one of the most common malignancies in industrialized societies, yet it is not well understood in the community at large. We believe that it is time to provide a simple, nonmedical explanation of this disease for people who have to deal with this illness either as patients or as caregivers.

Cancer can affect any part of the bladder. When bladder cancer is examined under a microscope, different types can be identified. Transitional cell cancer, which accounts for more than 90 percent of bladder cancers, begins in the innermost layer of bladder tissue and consists of cells of variable sizes and shapes. It is called "transitional" because it resembles some of the other patterns of cells that are found in bladder cancer and has been thought to be intermediate or transitional between some of them. Because of where it begins, it is also called urothelial cancer. Another pattern is squamous cell carcinoma, which starts in the flat cells that line the inside of the bladder and (under the microscope) closely resembles the appearance of the cells that make up the layers of skin. Adenocarcinoma begins in cells that have a glandlike appearance and make mucus. Squamous cell carcinoma and adenocarcinoma are very uncommon.

Cancer is not one disease; it is many diseases affecting parts of the human body. All cancers have one thing in common: Something has gone wrong in the way some of the body's cells normally grow, divide, and die. When a cancer forms, the main problem is that some cells start to grow, slowly or quickly, in an uncontrolled fashion, and the usual switch-off mechanisms that stop cell growth don't work properly. The breakdown in the switch-off mechanisms may be caused by exposure to chemicals (for example, some of those found in cigarette smoke), radiation, or even rare types of virus infection. The extra cells may cluster and form a tumor. Cancer cells may invade and damage surrounding tissue. Cancer cells may also break away and spread through the body by entering the lymph or blood systems. Most bladder cancers are treatable by techniques that kill them or remove them surgically as they sit on the inner surface of the bladder; others are invasive (having burrowed into the wall of the bladder) or metastatic (having spread to other parts of the body), and treatment is thus more complicated, as the following chapters will describe.

Bladder cancer primarily affects those between the ages of 50 and 70, more often men than women, and more Caucasians than African Americans, Hispanics, or Asians. Smokers, ex-smokers, and those who have jobs that expose them to certain chemicals or environmental toxins are at high risk of developing bladder cancer. Family members of those who have had bladder cancer are at *slightly* higher risk of developing the disease, and if you have already had bladder cancer, you have an increased chance of getting it again.

In this book we'll look at all aspects of bladder cancer and what you can expect each step of the way. We'll talk about symptoms, tests, diagnoses, treatments, recurrence probabilities, clinical trials, drug treatments, support groups, questions you'll want to ask your doctor, and how to deal with hospitals, insurance companies … and yes, even doctors.

Most important, we'll help you understand bladder cancer and how it might affect your life or that of a loved one, and we'll explore the resources available to you as you continue your journey.

Derek Raghavan, M.D., Ph.D.
Kathleen Tuthill

Chapter 1

The Bladder

The bladder is a balloon-shaped, muscular organ tucked into the pelvis and held in place by fibrous bands and muscle. The bladder is part of a system that includes the kidneys, ureters, and urethra. These work to process the waste products left behind after your body has taken out the nutrients it needs from the food you eat.

The bladder is lined on the inside by a tissue known as "urothelium," the smooth layer that stretches as the bladder fills and prevents excreted material from being reabsorbed into the body. Underneath the urothelium is a mix of fibrous or supporting tissue and muscle, both of which help the bladder to expand (when full) and to contract and excrete urine at the appropriate time.

Not only does the urothelium line the bladder; it also is found as the lining tissue elsewhere in the urinary tract system, including in the ureters (the tubes that drain the kidneys), the urethra (the tube that drains urine from the bladder to the exterior of the body), and parts of the male prostate. Urothelial tissue, too, can sometimes develop cancerous changes known as urothelial malignancy. The most common type of urothelial malignancy is "transitional cell carcinoma." (See Chapter 3.)

It's important to note that when the urothelial tissue is exposed to cancer-causing substances, such as the breakdown products of cigarette smoke, the potential exists for cancerous changes to occur in multiple areas. That's why when bladder cancer is suspected or confirmed, the whole urinary tract is screened for the possible presence of other cancerous deposits.

Other organs, such as the lungs, liver, skin, and intestinal tract, also process waste. These systems work together to balance the chemicals and water that your body needs to function properly.

The urinary system processes urea, a specific waste product that is produced when protein-containing foods (such as a meat) are broken down in the digestive process.

Urea is filtered through the kidneys and together with other waste by-products and water, becomes urine. This is carried by thin tubes called ureters to the bladder, where it is stored. Muscles in the walls of the ureters squeeze out small amounts of urine into the bladder on a constant basis, about every 10 seconds. A healthy bladder can hold about two cups of urine for up to five hours. Healthy adults produce about six cups of urine a day.

A strong muscle somewhat like a rubber band circles your bladder and keeps the urethra tightly closed until nerves in the bladder signal you that the bladder is full and it is time to urinate. Urinary problems include the inability to retain the urine in the normal fashion or to void urine from the body. Sometimes people experience the urge to urinate even if the bladder is not full. Sometimes this is caused by bacteria in the bladder, which can cause an infection called cystitis. This symptom can also be caused by local bladder irritation or by the development of cancer. As with all parts of the human body, the bladder can develop cancer, which can also cause problems with retaining or voiding urine.

SYMPTOMS

The most common symptom of bladder cancer is hematuria, or blood visible in the urine, either with or without any accompanying pain. About 85 percent of the people diagnosed with bladder cancer notice blood in their urine, and it's often what prompts them to seek medical attention.

In some cases, the presence of blood isn't noticeable to the naked eye and can only be seen through a microscope, usually when a urine test is being done during a routine physical or when an infection of the urinary tract or bladder is suspected. A urine test can detect whether blood is present in the urine and can also rule out whether other things, such as food or medicines, are the cause of red or rusty-colored urine.

Female urogenital system

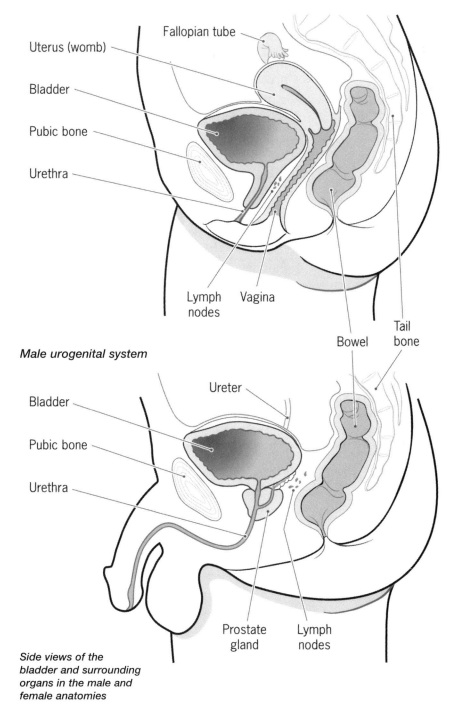

Side views of the bladder and surrounding organs in the male and female anatomies

Noticeable blood in the urine is a tricky symptom. It appears in varying colors and at irregular intervals, and as a result, you might overlook its significance or decide to wait and see whether it happens again before checking it out.

For example, you may notice blood in your urine or drops of blood in your underwear two or three times in as many days, or you may see it on one occasion but after that your urine appears normal for days or weeks. The same thing can happen with a laboratory urinalysis, where red blood cells may be visible microscopically only intermittently.

You might experience a gush of bright red blood or notice pink or rusty brown urine or even little clots of blood. To complicate things even more, foods you eat such as beets or blackberries may produce colored urine, as do a number of medicines, food additives, and vitamins.

With the major symptoms of bladder cancer acting in such a variable fashion, appearing in different ways and sometimes disappearing altogether, it's important to see your doctor immediately if you notice blood or what you think might be blood in your urine. As with most cancers, the key to successfully managing bladder cancer is detecting it early and starting treatment as soon as possible.

Bladder cancer does not have a long list of symptoms, and many of the symptoms are typical of other, less severe conditions such as infections or benign tumors. Besides blood in the urine, your symptoms can include pain or burning during urination, a feeling of having to urinate because of an uncomfortable fullness, or the need to get up frequently at night to urinate.

You may also have symptoms such as backache, abdominal pain, and unplanned weight loss, or you may feel more tired and achy than usual.

WHO GETS BLADDER CANCER?

The most significant factors that put you at high risk of developing bladder cancer are age, sex, history of exposure to cigarette smoke, and occupation.

Men are at much higher risk for bladder cancer than women, although it's not known why; it strikes men three to four times as often as it does women. However, recent statistics show that the disease appears to be rising among women.

Bladder cancer is the fourth most common cancer among men in the United States (following prostate, lung, and colon cancers) and the tenth most common cancer among women. It is most common in people between the ages of 50 and 70, and is rarely diagnosed in children.

While the incidence of bladder cancer in men has decreased since 1990, the decline follows a 50 percent increase in the disease since the 1960s.

Caucasians constitute the highest risk group. For reasons that are not yet known, fewer Asians develop bladder cancer, and African Americans have the lowest rate of all. The lifetime risk of developing bladder cancer is 2.8 percent for white men and 0.9 percent for African American men, and 1.0 percent for white women, compared to 0.6 percent for African American women.

Schistosomiasis, a parasite common in some Middle Eastern countries (particularly Egypt), is linked to a type of bladder cancer known as squamous cell carcinoma. The parasite isn't picked up by casual visitors, but instead may affect those who have traveled there for long periods or lived in the Middle East for any length of time. This latter group is at higher risk for *schistosomiasis* and its subsequent chronic irritation of the bladder, which can eventually result in tumors.

Most significant in the list of risk factors is exposure to cigarette smoke. It is estimated that up to 80 percent of all bladder cancers can be attributed to cigarette smoking, your own or possibly even someone else's, if you were nearby to inhale it ("passive smoking" or "secondhand smoke").

BLADDER CANCER BY THE NUMBERS

Caucasians constitute the highest risk group. For reasons that are not yet known, fewer Asians develop bladder cancer, and African Americans have the lowest rate of all. National Cancer Institute statistics from 2002 to 2004 show that lifetime risk of developing bladder cancer is 2.35 percent for all races. Among whites, the lifetime risk of developing bladder cancer is 2.55 percent, and among African Americans it is 1.13 percent.

From 2000-2004, incidence rates per 100,000 population:

	Men	Women		Men	Women
All Races	**37.3**	**9.4**			
White	40.5	10.1	American Indian/		
Black	20.3	7.6	Native Alaskan	11.9	3.2
Asian/Pacific	16.4	3.9	Hispanic	20.2	5.5

From 2000-2004, mortality rates per 100,000 population:

	Men	Women		Men	Women
All Races	**7.5**	**2.3**			
White	7.9	2.3	American Indian/		
Black	5.3	2.8	Native Alaskan	3.1	1.1
Asian/Pacific	2.9	1.0	Hispanic	3.9	1.4

Relative survival rate over 5 years, based on 1996-2004 figures:

White male	81.4 percent	White female	76.6 percent
Black male	68.2 percent	Black female	55.5 percent

Lifetime risk of developing bladder cancer between ages 50-70 based on rates from 2002-2004:

Men	1.22 percent	Women	0.35 percent

If you were raised by smokers or live in a house with smokers, you may be at risk, as are those who are current or former smokers. To a lesser extent, smoking pipes or cigars also carries a risk. Snuff and chewing tobacco have not been linked to bladder cancer.

The risk of bladder cancer quickly drops when you quit smoking. However, as an ex-smoker you remain at risk because it can take 20 or 30 years for bladder cancer to manifest itself. Certain variables, such as how deeply you inhaled cigarette smoke and how long you smoked, can elevate or reduce your risk.

Occupational exposure to certain chemicals accounts for up to 20 percent of bladder cancers. Some of those chemicals, such as the benzidine used in the textile dye and rubber-tire industries, have been banned in the workplace. Other suspected carcinogens (cancer-causing substances), such as 4-nitrobiphenyl, 2-naphthylamine, and 4-aminobiphenyl, are still in use, however, and have led to some occupations being earmarked as high or moderate risk for bladder cancer. Workers at risk among those occupations include:

- Laborers in textile dye, rubber, and chemical industries with exposure to aromatic amines
- Some pharmaceutical or pesticide manufacturers
- Workers employed in coal or gas production
- Painters
- Truck drivers
- Hairdressers
- Sewage workers
- Metalworkers in the aluminum, iron, and steel industries

Other risk factors include chronic urinary tract infections, exposure to cyclophosphamide or ifosfamide (chemotherapy drugs used for certain cancers), and pelvic radiation for cervical cancer. Also, there is a somewhat elevated chance of your developing bladder cancer if a member of your family has had the disease. Although there is evidence that saccharin consumption is a risk factor, various studies have failed to find a strong link between caffeine and modern artificial sweeteners. People who consume lots of fluids have been reported to have a lower incidence of bladder cancer, perhaps because fluids flush cancer-causing chemicals out of the bladder.

The most recent cancer research indicates that bladder cancer might be prevented through changes in lifestyle, so don't use tobacco products and be sure to limit your exposure to certain chemicals, drugs, and radiation.

Some risk factors, such as heredity, can't be controlled, but you can be aware of them and of any symptoms of diseases that have appeared in previous generations of your family. Do keep in mind that even if an inheritable disease is present in your family history, it doesn't mean that everyone in your family will actually *get* the disease. In fact, most won't. But because you have an increased *likelihood* of developing the disease, you can and should get regular checkups so that if cancer does develop, you'll catch it early, at a stage when treatment is most effective.

DIAGNOSIS CASE STUDY: MAX, AGE 62

Max was worried when he noticed that his urine was rusty brown one morning, but he put off doing anything about it at first. He still worked part-time at Maple Grove's water-treatment plant, and the EPA was due any day to make its annual inspection. He needed to be there, keeping tabs on his crews and making sure that there were no glitches when the EPA team arrived.

Besides, everything was fine the next time Max went to the bathroom. Normal. Yellow. It didn't hurt when he urinated, although it did burn a little sometimes and he found himself getting up four or five times a night to go to the bathroom. He chalked that up to getting older, though.

But when the rusty brown urine appeared again a few days later, he told his wife, Jean, who immediately called the doctor's office. The nurse told Max to take a urine sample to the lab the next morning and made an office appointment for two days after that.

When Max came in to see Dr. J, the nurse asked him a number of questions. When did the symptoms start? How would he describe the color of the urine? Were there any clots of blood visible? Any pain when he urinated? Had he ever had blood in his urine before? Did he have any itching or burning? Any fever?

She performed the usual blood-pressure check, declaring it "perfect," and left his file, complete with her notes from the questions she asked Max, tucked into the holder on the front of the examining-room door.

Blood in his urine? Max immediately jumped to the conclusion that the nurse had seen the urine-test results and knew it was blood. Max had suspected as much but hearing it out loud … well, that was scary.

Dr. J came in and asked the same questions the nurse had, plus a few more. Was he getting up frequently at night to urinate? Did his bladder feel full, even when he didn't have to urinate? Had he had any unplanned weight loss? A cough?

Max, who was feeling very anxious by now about what might be wrong with him, lashed out at Dr. J.

"You know, I just answered these questions for your nurse. Doesn't any one here write things down? Or read what does get written down?"

Dr. J smiled. "Max, doctors are trained to get information right from the source – the patient – even if there are detailed notes made by a nurse or another doctor. It's easy to make a wrong assumption or to misinterpret someone else's information, and that could adversely affect my diagnosis or treatment plan for you. I guess from your point of view, it seems as if we don't communicate. But really, we're just trying to get it right."

Max nodded. "Okay. I can understand that. It just seems sometimes that the same things are asked over and over, and it gets frustrating." Feeling calmer, he added, "What else do you want to know, Doc?"

"How about smoking? You quit a few years ago, didn't you?"

Max admitted that he still smoked a few cigarettes a day, although not in his house. His wife wouldn't let him.

"Good for her. Smoking or living with a cigarette smoker puts you *and* her at risk for all kinds of health problems. I want you to get serious about quitting, Max. Very serious."

Dr. J performed a physical exam and then told Max to get dressed and come down his office to talk. Max didn't like the sound of that.

URINALYSIS: THREE CATEGORIES

Routine urinalysis examines the urine. It falls into three categories: macroscopic, dipstick, and microscopic.

Macroscopic Urinalysis

Macroscopic Urinalysis is simply visual observation of the color and clarity (or cloudiness) of the urine.

Dipsticks

Dipsticks are plastic or paper "sticks" coated with chemicals that change color if certain substances (such as glucose, protein, or blood) are present in the urine. Dipsticks provide immediate results and are cost-effective, but they provide limited information. For example, a dipstick test can confirm the presence of protein in the urine, but it doesn't measure the quantity. More accurate measurements can be made on collected urine by a chemical analyzer, a machine that can measure the presence of sugar, protein, or other substances in the urine.

Microscopic Urinalysis

For detailed analysis of the cells present in urine, a microscopic urinalysis is performed. For this test, urine is prepared in a laboratory – usually by being spun in a centrifuge – and examined under a microscope for blood cells, cancer cells, or bacteria.

To prepare for a urinalysis, you should avoid heavy athletic activity or physical labor the day before the test, since this activity can sometimes result in the appearance of small amounts of blood in the urine. Collect the urine first thing in the morning, if possible, using a sterile, covered container. (This is usually provided by the doctor's office or laboratory.) Thoroughly wash the area around the urethra (the body opening where urine exits the body). Let the first few drops of urine fall into the toilet; this clears the urethra of any remaining contaminants. Catch a few ounces of urine in the clean container, and if you are not able to give it immediately to a nurse or laboratory assistant, store the urine in a cool place. (Your refrigerator is fine.) Make sure you get the urine sample to the doctor's office or laboratory within four hours.

At times, your doctor may want to use a catheter (a thin, flexible tube) to take a urine specimen directly from the bladder. This can be done in your doctor's office with a minimum of discomfort. Your doctor will use a local anesthetic cream to numb the tip of the penis and, in both men and women, the urethra.

Some medications discolor or cause false results in a urinalysis. Make sure your doctor has a list of all medications you take regularly, including over-the-counter antacids or pain relievers, vitamins, calcium and other minerals, and herbal supplements or teas.

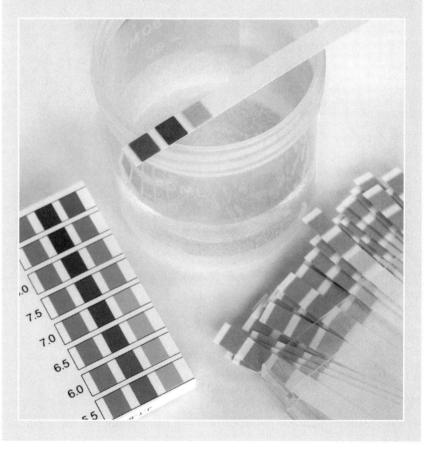

Dr. J usually talked to him right there in the examining room. He threw on his clothes and hurried down the hall.

"Max, I want you to see a urologist at the Glickman Urological and Kidney Institute at Cleveland Clinic. The results of the urine test show some red blood cells in your urine, and given what you've told me today about your symptoms and history, I think further tests are in order to rule out certain conditions. I'm more comfortable having him do those tests."

"So what do you think the problem is?" Max asked. "Something with my kidneys?"

"I think more likely it's bladder disease, Max."

"Like an infection or something?"

"That's possible, but I don't think it's very likely. We need to rule out a few things. This could be a benign condition, such as an infection, or it could be bladder cancer. I know that's a scary thing to hear, but there are lots of red flags that put you in a high-risk category. Your age, sex, occupation, symptoms, smoking. If it is bladder cancer, Max – and right now we don't know that it is – the sooner we treat it, the better."

Dr. J explained that there were some tests the urologist would want to do and gave Max a pamphlet about bladder cancer and how it's diagnosed.

"I know it's easier said than done, but don't start worrying yet, Max. The urologist will eliminate the possible causes of the red blood cells in your urine, and we'll go from there. Let's see what the tests show."

For a brief moment, Max wished that Jean hadn't called Dr. J. Then he wouldn't have heard the words "bladder cancer" and wouldn't be feeling sick to his stomach. What would having cancer be like? Would he have surgery? Chemotherapy?

Max took a deep breath. "Okay, I guess I'd better go see the urologist."

At the Urologist's Office

The urologist scheduled an ultrasound and intravenous pyelography (IVP). He told Max that depending on the results, he might schedule more tests.

Max had the IVP test first. He grumbled about having to fast in the morning and grumbled even more about the laxative he had to take the night before.

The test itself, he admitted, was a breeze. Other than a pinprick from the needle for the IV and a nasty metallic taste in his mouth while the x-rays were being taken, it was, according to Max, "a piece of cake. Not like that ultrasound. I thought I'd burst."

For the ultrasound, Max had had to drink a large amount of liquid so that his bladder would be full during the test; this made it easier to get a good reading. The test itself hadn't been painful or unpleasant – once he'd been able to go the bathroom and void all that fluid!

It took two weeks before the tests were done and the results in the doctor's hands. Max spent many a sleepless night worrying. Most of the time he could be optimistic about his future, even if the verdict was cancer. But in the middle of the night, when Jean was sleeping and the house was quiet, Max got scared, deep down, gut-level scared. *What if it is cancer? What if I'm going to die?*

Finally, the time came for Max and Jean to go to the doctor's office. He told them that Max did, indeed, have bladder cancer, but that the tumor was limited to the surface of the bladder (he called it "superficial") and noninvasive.

Hearing the words "superficial tumor" and "noninvasive," Max let out a sigh of relief. He had convinced himself that the news would be more serious.

The doctor explained that Max's tumor was confined to the transitional cell epithelium. Treatment, he said, would consist of a small surgical procedure (a "resection") to remove the tumor, followed by a series of bladder washes through a urinary catheter, using an immunological treatment called Bacille Calmette-Guérin, or BCG, to help make sure the cancer didn't recur. Max turned to Jean and said, "Well, looks like you're stuck with me another few years."

"I can deal with that," said Jean, the tears trickling down her cheeks.

The doctor cautioned Max and Jean that the word "superficial" wasn't interchangeable with "harmless."

"Superficial TCC is highly treatable, but it has a high recurrence rate, Max. Sometimes when it recurs it is at a more serious level. I don't want to alarm you, as there is every reason to expect a good outcome in your case, but I do want you to be aware of the possibilities and to impress upon you the importance of follow-up."

The urologist continued, "If your cancer does come back, it's likely to be during the first two years, so we're going to keep a close eye on you, Max. We'll do urine tests and flexible cystoscopies regularly. And I want to know right away if you have any symptoms like blood in your urine or painful urination, or if you're more tired than usual or have any new aches or pains, or a persistent cough."

Max was still floating on the hopefulness of his diagnosis. It was Jean who answered. "Don't worry, I'll keep him honest." ◆

SMOKING-CESSATION RESOURCES

- The **American Cancer Society** sponsors the Great American Smokeout each November and makes resources about quitting smoking available at www.cancer.org. You can also call 1-800-227-2345 (1-800-ACS-2345) for information. (Check your phone book for your local American Cancer Society office.)

- **The American Heart Association** makes available books, tapes, and videos about quitting smoking. Information can be found at www.americanheart.org or by calling 1-800-242-8721. (Check your phone book for your local American Heart Association office.)

- **The American Lung Association** offers a self-help quit program called Freedom from Smoking. Find information about Freedom from Smoking at www.lungusa.org or by calling 1-800-LUNG-USA (1-800-586-4872). (For local American Lung Association offices check your phone book.)

- **Ask your doctor** about the advisability of using over-the-counter or prescription nicotine patches, gums, and other treatments as part of your program to stop smoking. Also ask for help locating local groups that sponsor smoking-cessation programs or support groups.

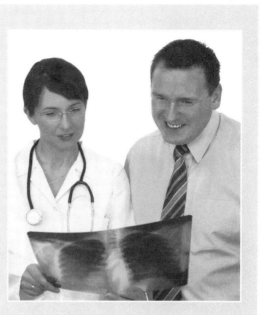

- **Cleveland Clinic** has been very active in promoting smoking cessation and has been completely smoke-free since July 4, 2005. In addition, it provides smoking-cessation programs and assistance for patients and staff. Information is available at www.clevelandclinic.org/smashtheash.

- **The National Cancer Institute** website at www.cancer.gov provides a link to information about quitting (www.smokefree.gov). It also has a telephone quitline (1-877-448-7848). Live help with questions or problems about quitting smoking is available at the NCI website by clicking on the LiveHelp link at www.cancer.gov.

- ***Stop Smoking Now! A Cleveland Clinic Guide,*** by Garland Y. DeNelsky, Ph.D., founder of the Clinic's smoking-cessation programs, details an approach to quitting smoking that has proved effective for countless smokers over the years. It can be ordered at www.clevelandclinicpress.org, www.amazon.com, and www.barnesandnoble.com.

Chapter 2

Diagnosis and Tests

DIAGNOSING BLADDER CANCER

After taking a history and performing a physical examination, among the first steps most physicians take in diagnosing bladder cancer are a urinalysis and some or all of the following tests: intravenous pyelography (IVP), an ultrasound, and x-rays, followed by a flexible cystoscopy. These tests are discussed later in this chapter.

Typically the IVP and ultrasound are the first steps in the diagnostic process. However, in some circumstances, doctors prefer to perform the flexible cystoscopy first.

Sometimes your family doctor will schedule these tests (although it is the urologist who performs a cystoscopy, if needed); sometimes your doctor will refer you to a urologist for all the tests. It's not important from your standpoint whether the urologist or family doctor does the tests, so long as the tests are completed.

UROLOGISTS AT CLEVELAND CLINIC

Most family doctors or internists will refer you to a urologist at some point in the initial diagnostic process. At Cleveland Clinic's Glickman Urological and Kidney Institute, the urologists are highly trained specialists who are experienced in the treatment of urinary tract disease, including bladder cancer. Usually board-certified and licensed in the urology field, these doctors are up to date in the latest diagnostic and treatment methods. The Glickman Urological and Kidney Institute is ranked No. 2 in the United States and has been a top urological center for many years.

It's also important to note that the experience does not unfold in exactly the same order for all people during the diagnostic progression. Which tests are ordered and when they are performed will depend to some degree on the results of each previous test. Besides the tests mentioned above, some or all of the following procedures may also be used in the diagnostic process: a CAT or CT scan, an MRI scan, an inpatient or outpatient cystoscopy, and surgical biopsy. (Each of these procedures will be discussed in this chapter.)

WHAT TO EXPECT DURING THE INITIAL DIAGNOSTIC PROCESS

If you have gone to your doctor complaining about any of the symptoms described in Chapter 1, your doctor will take a detailed history and perform a full physical examination, and will probably schedule a urinalysis and perhaps additional tests.

During your office visit, your doctor will ask you detailed questions about your lifestyle, symptoms, and medical history. Your doctor may ask you questions that don't seem relevant to your symptoms, such as whether you have abdominal pain or your bones ache more than usual, and whether you've unexpectedly lost weight or developed a cough. The doctor is looking for indications that cancer might be present elsewhere in the body; such indications will determine what tests to recommend.

Routine body functions such as lung, heart, and blood pressure should be checked. Your abdomen should be examined, and for men, a prostate exam should be performed, while women should expect a vaginal exam.

At this point, the doctor may schedule further tests or refer you to a urologist.

The descriptions included here of procedures and test processes or preparations are of a general nature; your experience during your actual process, preparation, or procedure may differ from what is discussed here.

Flexible Cystoscopy

When you are referred to a urologist, he, too, will take a history and perform a careful physical examination. He may then suggest a flexible cystoscopy. This is a procedure that allows the urologist to look around inside your bladder for the presence of small tumors or abnormalities without doing an invasive, or surgical, procedure. Flexible cystoscopy is usually performed in your physician's office under local anesthetic, although in some cases, it's preferable to conduct a similar procedure, called a rigid cystoscopy, under general anesthesia in a hospital setting.

Cancer has the potential to arise at any part of the urothelial tract (the lining of the bladder, ureters, etc.), so the urologist will carefully examine the whole of the bladder and will sometimes use a different scope – one with a smaller gauge – called a ureteroscope to examine the upper urinary tracts (ureters). This is not a painful procedure and is simply an extension of the cystoscopy, using a slightly different gadget.

If your doctor scheduled an IVP first and tumors were observed, the flexible cystoscopy test may be omitted and other tests may be recommended for you as the next step in the diagnostic process.

During the flexible cystoscopy, a thin flexible tube with a lighted lens or fiber optic is inserted into your bladder through the urethra. To minimize pain, a local anesthetic in the form of a cream or gel is gently applied in the urethra first. A sterile liquid, usually a saline solution, flows through the cystoscope, filling and stretching your bladder. You may feel some fullness and the urge to urinate during a

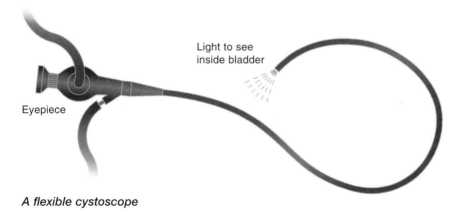

Light to see
inside bladder

Eyepiece

A flexible cystoscope

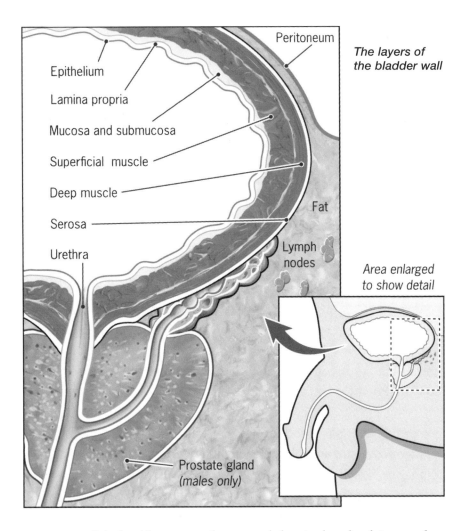

*The layers of
the bladder wall*

Peritoneum

Epithelium

Lamina propria

Mucosa and submucosa

Superficial muscle

Deep muscle

Serosa

Urethra

Fat

Lymph
nodes

*Area enlarged
to show detail*

Prostate gland
(males only)

cystoscopy. It helps if you can relax your abdominal and pelvic muscles.

Through a lens or on a screen, your doctor watches the images transmitted from the bladder by the cystoscope. Sometimes urine that is in your bladder at the time of cystoscopy will be collected for examination, or a tissue sample may be taken for biopsy.

Your doctor will also digitally examine your bladder with a gloved finger, from the rectum if you're a man and also from the vagina if you're a woman, to determine whether there is any thickening of your bladder wall, which can be an indication of an invasive tumor. Pressing gently with the finger, the doctor can feel abnormalities in the wall or position of the bladder.

Patients sometimes describe feeling some abdominal pressure or discomfort, but not pain, during the flexible cystoscopy procedure. You will be awake, wearing a gown and lying on an examining table, with your knees draped and held apart. As noted above, your doctor will use anesthetic gel to numb the area where the flexible tube is inserted and then gently guide the cystoscope into the urethral opening (the eye of the penis in a man; the vaginal outlet of the urethra in a woman). Some men experience brief pressure and discomfort as the cystoscope passes over the area where the prostate is located.

In most cases, the entire process, including preparation, will take about 15 to 20 minutes, and your doctor will be able to discuss the results of the flexible cystoscopy with you immediately.

Rigid Cystoscopy

The rigid cystoscopy is sometimes done when the tumor is in an inaccessible part of the bladder as well as when a more complicated biopsy is needed. It is performed in a hospital setting and can be either an inpatient or outpatient procedure. While the process is similar to flexible cystoscopy, you will be given general anesthesia and a more rigid tube will be used.

Your doctor will give you specific instructions about how to prepare for the anesthesia (you will need to have someone drive you to and from the hospital) and what to expect during the brief recuperation after the procedure. You may be asked to remain overnight if you have other medical problems, such as severe heart disease.

Intravenous Pyelography (IVP)

Intravenous pyelography is a form of x-ray. It is painless except for the pinprick from the intravenous needle. The IVP test (and all of the following x-ray or scan procedures) are performed by a radiologist and radiology technologists at your hospital's radiology department or at a recommended imaging center.

The IVP helps physicians see most cysts, stones, abnormalities, or tumors in the bladder. Because small tumors don't show up on an IVP but may be visible during a flexible cystoscopy, often both procedures are used as diagnostic tools.

During the IVP, you'll be lying on a flat table, wearing a hospital gown, with the x-ray machine positioned above you on a movable jointed arm.

The radiologist will take some basic x-rays and then will inject a contrast substance (usually iodine) through a vein, usually in your arm. The iodine is carried by the blood system to the kidneys, where it is removed (excreted into the urine). The iodine shows up when exposed in an x-ray.

You might feel a sense of heat or burning from the iodine or have a metallic taste in your mouth. However, these sensations usually disappear after a few minutes. If you know that you are allergic to iodine, let the radiologist know and a different contrast material can be used.

As the iodine travels through your urinary tract system, a quick series of x-rays is snapped. Sometimes the radiologist will apply a gentle compression elastic band around your body to help the visualization process. You may be asked to turn over and might even be asked to empty your bladder. (The iodine should not cause any discoloration of your urine or any pain or burning during urination.)

The x-rays taken before the iodine was injected and those taken after provide images for your doctor that give a visual picture of the ureters (the tubes between the kidneys and bladder) and the bladder's anatomy and function.

Ultrasound

Your doctor may also recommend an ultrasound, sometimes called a sonogram, to help examine your bladder.

An ultrasound, as its name suggests, is an imaging process that uses high-frequency sound waves that bounce off organs such as the bladder to create a visible image. It's a painless, very safe procedure that usually takes less than half an hour to complete.

You'll be lying down on an examining table, wearing a gown and covered by a drape. A technologist will smear a clear gel over your abdomen. This often feels clammy and cold, but it's necessary to help transmit the sound waves.

The technologist then moves a transducer (an imaging gadget shaped somewhat like an oversized electric shaver with a flat head) over the area where the bladder is located. You probably will be asked to change positions or even to hold your breath for a few seconds during the process. The technologist watches on a screen to make sure that clear images are being recorded.

THE NEXT STEP IN THE DIAGNOSTIC PROCESS

If any of the tests suggest the presence of a bladder tumor, your doctor will schedule other tests; they might include an MRI or a CT scan, and if a biopsy was not obtained during the flexible cystoscopy process, a surgical biopsy as well. These tests help your doctor determine where the tumors are, what type of cancer you have, and whether the cancer has invaded the muscle wall of the bladder. Depending on the results of those tests, your doctor may order a chest x-ray or even a bone scan to determine whether the cancer has spread to other areas of the body.

Computed Tomography (CT or CAT Scan)

A CT scan is a painless, noninvasive test during which low intensity x-rays are repeatedly passed through the body's soft tissue at different angles. A computer then processes the x-rays to show a detailed cross-section of the tissues and organs – in your case, of the bladder, liver, spleen, abdominal lymph nodes, and surrounding tissues. Sometimes the scanner will be focused on the chest and lungs to see whether cancer has spread there.

From the CT scan, your doctor not only can confirm the presence of a tumor in the bladder, but can also measure its size and location, and determine whether it has spread to other nearby tissue.

The CT scanner is a large rectangular machine with an opening for an x-ray "tube" that will move around your body, snapping "pictures" that the computer will assemble into a set of cross-section scans that can be viewed by the physician. These scans show remarkably clear images of the various organs. The scanner usually makes a whirring sound as it moves and a click similar to a camera as it snaps images.

The CT scanner can snap about 32 cross-section pictures or "slices" in approximately 10 seconds as the machine moves over your body. This means that you can easily hold your breath as the images are taken.

For the CT scan, you'll be lying on a table, dressed in a gown, and while you'll be able to talk with the radiology technicians at all times over an intercom, you'll be alone in the room and asked to lie still and hold your breath while the actual x-rays are being taken.

Like the IVP, a contrast medium is used to help the radiologist see your bladder and urinary tract. Sometimes it may be injected into the veins, as in IVP, or it may be swallowed or sometimes administered as an enema to distinguish bowel tissue from the bladder structure. Usually when diagnosing bladder cancer, doctors will want all three – intravenous, oral, and rectal scans – to help determine how deeply tumors may have invaded the bladder tissue and whether there is any spread to the abdominal lymph nodes or liver.

Some people find the taste of the contrast medium unpleasant, and if an enema is required, you're likely to feel a brief, uncomfortable fullness while the scans are being taken. However, because of the speed of the process, the feeling that you need to expel the contrast medium doesn't last long. You might also feel a brief flush or hot sensation when the contrast medium is injected.

A CT scan takes anywhere from 5 to 30 minutes. Other than mild discomfort, there are few side effects.

Nuclear Magnetic Resonance Imaging (NMR or MRI) Scan

Sometimes doctors prefer to use an MRI instead of a CT scan. Like the CT scan, an MRI is painless and noninvasive, but unlike the CT scan, no radiation is involved. An MRI uses radiofrequency waves and an electromagnetic field to stimulate atomic nuclei in the body. The energy released by these nuclei is recorded and provides an accurate visualization of soft tissue in your body.

A Magnetic Resonance Imaging (MRI) machine

The MRI machine is a big metal box with a tunnel through its middle and a narrow sliding table. You'll lie on the sliding table, which will move you slowly through the electromagnetic field or "tunnel" of the MRI machine. An MRI can take anywhere from 15 to 45 minutes. Some MRI machines are closed cylinders; others have wider tunnels and open sides to reduce the claustrophobic feelings that some people experience. If you suffer from claustrophobia – the fear of close or enclosed spaces – you should warn your doctor that you might not be comfortable having an MRI scan.

You'll wear a gown, and as with the CT scan, the radiology technicians leave the room during the scanning process, but you'll be able to communicate with them through an intercom. Sometimes a friend or relative is permitted to sit in the room with you, particularly if you are claustrophobic. Sometimes if you are claustrophobic a gentle sedative is used to help you to feel comfortable in the machine.

Sometimes a contrast medium is used, usually intravenous, in which case you might experience a cool sensation. You'll be asked to remain very still for short periods while the images are being taken, usually anywhere from a few seconds to a few minutes at a time. You'll be able to move slightly between "takes" or images.

Other than what many patients describe as a "closed-in" feeling, the single most uncomfortable part of an MRI is not being able to move about. Sometimes you'll also hear a banging sound as the scans are being taken. This can be surprisingly noisy. Many physicians feel that the MRI scanner is a useful alternative to the CT scanner, but results can be more difficult to interpret when the MRI scan is focused on the back of the abdomen, the pelvis, and bladder, so generally CT scans are more frequently used.

Surgical Biopsy

Usually performed under general anesthesia in a hospital, a biopsy via a rigid cystoscope allows the physician to examine your bladder manually for any abnormalities (again, by inserting a finger into the rectum and feeling the local tissues) and then to remove small amounts of tissue. These can then be examined microscopically and used to confirm the presence of cancer and the invasiveness of the disease, as well as to help determine the appropriate treatment.

Sometimes, in the case of small or superficial tumors, the physician will remove the entire tumor and surrounding tissue for biopsy. As with all surgeries or invasive procedures, a biopsy may involve some pain as well as a brief recovery time that might call for some limitations on physical activities for a day or two. The urologist will prescribe pain-relieving medication to reduce the severity of discomfort.

Other Tests

If your test results suggest that the cancer may have spread to other organs or areas of the body, your doctor may schedule a chest x-ray or bone scan.

GETTING A SECOND OPINION

You may want a second opinion about your diagnosis. In fact, some insurance companies require you to get a second opinion, even though you might be worried about delaying your treatment. Don't be. A brief delay while you gather your records and talk to another doctor or medical team shouldn't prove to be a problem.

How do you go about finding another doctor for a second opinion?

- First, you might ask your doctor for a recommendation to another expert who can give a second opinion.

- You can call 1-800-422-6237 (1-800-4-CANCER) and the National Cancer Institute will tell you about treatment centers it supports.

- You can check with your local medical society, a nearby hospital, or even a medical college if one is nearby. Most states have NCI-designated Comprehensive Cancer Centers, and doctors at such institutions will usually provide a second opinion if requested.

- The American Board of Medical Specialists has a publication – *The Official ABMS Directory of Board Certified Medical Specialists* – that lists certified doctors, and the same list can be found at http://www.abms.org. (Click on "Is Your Doctor Certified?")

- In addition, there are two annual publications, *America's Top Doctors* (published by Castle Connolly; http://www.castleconnolly.com/books/index.cfm) and *Best 100 Doctors in America,* both of which list prominent cancer specialists whose peers have identified them as real experts. (The *Best 100 Doctors* list is compiled by BestDoctors.com, launched in 1989 by doctors affiliated with Harvard University. The list is not released to the general public. Instead, the annual list of *Best 100 Doctors* is provided to designated regional magazines and to hospitals. Check with the health center where you plan to receive treatment to find out which of its doctors may be included on this list.)

A **chest x-ray** is a type of x-ray process that takes about 10 minutes. You'll wear a gown and remain standing during the x-ray. The radiology technician will ask you to stand in several positions and will take x-rays of the chest area. It's a painless process and doesn't require that you inject or drink any contrast medium. This test can indicate whether the cancer has spread to the lungs and also can reveal other, unrelated medical conditions, such as a chest infection.

A **bone scan** uses a very small amount of a radioactive tracer injected into the bloodstream. Bone absorbs the tracer, which gives off gamma rays; these are then scanned to identify areas of abnormality. The purpose of this test is to monitor for the presence of cancer metastases in the bones, but it can also detect infection or arthritis sometimes.

It's a time-consuming test. It takes about three hours for the bone to absorb the tracer after it's injected into your vein (usually in an arm). What usually happens is that after the tracer is injected, you'll leave for a few hours or wait in the waiting room. (Bring a book.) The scan itself will take about an hour.

For the scan, you'll lie on a stationary table while a big cylinder – actually a gamma camera – moves up and down the table taking pictures. The cylinder doesn't enclose you to the extent that an MRI machine does and usually doesn't provoke a claustrophobic feeling. As with a CT or MRI scan, you'll lie on a table, wearing a gown, and will have to remain still when the gamma camera is clicking away, sometimes for several minutes at a time. You'll be asked to change positions several times during the scan, a welcome relief after you've had to remain motionless.

Sometimes tests on the urine are done to determine the presence of biomarkers. These are proteins that may be liberated by bladder-cancer cells into the urine. One example is the **NMP22** or **BladderCheck** test. For this, a few drops of voided urine are tested chemically on a glass slide. Some physicians believe that the NMP22 is more sensitive and more accurate than the more conventional cytology test, in which urine is examined for cancer cells under a microscope.

AFTER THE TESTS HAVE BEEN COMPLETED

Once your physician has gathered all the test results, they will be carefully evaluated by your doctor and the radiologist. In addition, your doctor may suggest bringing an oncologist on board your medical team at this point.

The next step will be for you and your family to discuss with the doctor what the tests and biopsy results mean, and to determine the course of treatment that is right for you.

If you had symptoms that suggest possible bladder cancer, make sure your physician checks you out thoroughly. If, for example, IVP results don't show the presence of any tumors, you'll want to go ahead and have a flexible cystoscopy and a CT scan or MRI to eliminate any possibility of abnormalities or carcinoma. If all tests are negative, generally no further follow-up is necessary unless your symptoms – particularly the painless passing of blood in the urine – occur again.

TESTS, RISKS, AND PRECAUTIONS

Here are some details about the tests your doctor may order.

Flexible Cystoscopy

This 30-minute test is performed in the doctor's office. You'll return home without assistance the same day. Discomfort is minimal.

Preparation: A local anesthetic, usually a gel, is applied before the procedure. You'll wear a hospital gown.

Risks: The test is generally safe. There is possibility of infection or bleeding; rarely, there is perforation of the bladder.

After effects: There may be burning during urination and a small amount of blood may be visible. If either continues after 24 hours (or if blood continues to appear after voiding has occurred three or more times), the doctor should be informed. When you're unable to urinate, the doctor should be contacted or you should go to a hospital emergency department. You should drink plenty of fluids.

Precautions: An allergic reaction to the sterile fluid or anesthetic gel is possible. If you're taking a blood-thinner, you must inform your doctor.

Rigid Cystoscopy

This surgical procedure is performed in the hospital while you're under general anesthesia (i.e., asleep). Recovery time is brief; if you're able to urinate, you'll go home the same day. (You'll need a driver.) You'll need rest for 24 hours and your activity will be restricted for a short time. Mild discomfort may limit some activities.

Preparation: Fasting is necessary, usually for a minimum of 12 hours prior to surgery. Antibiotics may be prescribed.

Risks: The procedure is generally safe. There is possibility of infection, difficulty urinating, bleeding, swelling, or (rarely) perforation. Occasionally, urinary retention occurs, requiring a catheter. Complications from anesthesia are possible.

After effects: Pain is minimal. Swelling or burning may occur during urination. (These reactions are normal.) Blood may appear in the urine occasionally for up to three weeks. You should call your doctor immediately if fever or excessive bleeding occurs, clots appear in the urine, testicular pain develops, or urination is not possible.

Precautions: If you're taking a blood-thinner, you must inform your doctor *before* the procedure.

Intravenous Pyelography (IVP)

This outpatient procedure is performed at an imaging center/hospital radiology center. It can take up to 60 minutes (possibly longer). It is noninvasive and discomfort is minimal.

Preparation: The test is preceded by a 12-hour fast. A laxative may be prescribed for the evening before the test. You'll wear a hospital gown. All jewelry or metal must be removed.

Risks: An allergic reaction to the contrast medium or iodine is possible. There is a very low risk of exposure to radiation.

After effects: You may experience a mild itching or hives may appear. If the condition persists, you should notify your doctor.

Precautions: If you're pregnant or nursing, inform your doctor. Tell your doctor about any allergies (especially to shellfish) that you may have. If you're diabetic, let your doctor know. And tell your doctor about any medications you are taking.

Ultrasound

This test is performed at an imaging center/hospital radiology center. It usually lasts less than 30 minutes. It is noninvasive, and any discomfort is very minimal.

Preparation: You'll have to fast for several hours before the test. Usually, you wear a hospital gown. An hour before the test, you must drink and retain four to six glasses of fluid.

Risks: There is a very low risk of allergic reaction to the conducting gel.

After effects: There are no after effects.

Precautions: If you have any allergies or have recently undergone a barium x-ray, your doctor should be informed.

Computed Tomography (CT or CAT Scan)

This test is performed on an outpatient basis at an imaging center/hospital radiology center. It usually takes 60 minutes or less, but it may last up to two hours. It is noninvasive and there is minimal discomfort. If you require a sedative, you will need to arrange to be driven home.

Preparation: Preparations can vary. A fast of up to 12 hours is usually called for. For some scans, you must take a laxative or enema the night before. You may need to have a blood test of kidney function in advance. You may be asked to drink a contrast solution before the test. You'll wear comfortable loose clothing (without zippers or snaps) or perhaps a hospital gown. All metal objects (such as jewelry, hairpins, dentures, and hearing aids) must be removed.

Risks: The test involves very low exposure to radiation. An allergic reaction (rarely serious) to the contrast material used in the test is possible.

After effects: During the test, you may feel warm or flushed, have a metallic taste in the mouth, or experience a headache or slight feeling of nausea. For 24 hours after the test, you should drink plenty of fluids.

Precautions: If there is any possibility that you may be pregnant, the doctor should be told. If you are nursing, you should wait 24 hours after the test before resuming. The doctor should be told if you have allergies (especially to iodine); are asthmatic; have problems with your kidneys, heart, or thyroid; have mutiple myeloma; or take metformin for diabetes.

Magnetic Resonance Imaging or Nuclear Magnetic Resonance Imaging (MRI)

This test is performed at an imaging center/hospital radiology center. It usually takes up to 60 minutes but may last as long as two hours. It is noninvasive. (However, an intravenous line may be used.) Discomfort is minimal, beyond the occasional discomfort at being confined. If you are claustrophobic, you should notify your doctors; you may require sedation or an open body-scan machine. If you're going to receive a sedative, you should arrange for a driver to take you home after the test.

Preparation: You'll wear comfortable loose clothing (without zippers or snaps) or perhaps a hospital gown. All metal objects (such as jewelry, hairpins, dentures, and hearing aids) must be removed. Some people prefer to bring earplugs or headphones to use during the test.

Risks: An undetected metal implant may react to the strong magnetic field. There is a low risk of allergic reaction to the contrast fluid used in the test.

After effects: If you have metal fillings in your teeth, you may feel a tingling in your mouth. Reactions during the test may include slight nausea, vomiting, headache, dizziness, pain, burning, or breathing problems.

Precautions: Let your doctor know if you have a prosthetic limb or hip; a pacemaker; an IUD; an artificial valve; an implanted port catheter; or any metal pins, plates, screws, or surgical staples in the body. Tell your doctor about any allergies or medical conditions you may have. If you are (or may be) pregnant or wear a medication patch, tell your doctor. If you're claustrophobic, let the doctor know when you schedule the test. And tell your doctor if you have any tattoos.

Surgical Biopsy

This is performed in association with cystoscopy. It can be done on an outpatient basis or as an overnight stay.

Preparation: Patients usually need to fast for several hours before the procedure, so check with your urologist when you schedule the test. Jewelry should be left at home.

Risks: The procedure is generally safe. You may have some lower abdominal pain post-biopsy and may note blood in your urine for a few days.

After effects: You may feel some burning during urination as well as post-biopsy discomfort or pain. Analgesics should be used as prescribed.

Precautions: The doctor should be told of persistent bleeding or pain or other unexpected symptoms. On rare occasions, an inability to pass urine may require a temporary urinary catheter.

Chest X-Ray

This test is performed at an imaging center/hospital radiology center. It usually takes about 10 minutes.

Preparation: You wear a hospital gown and must remove jewelry or metallic objects from the waist to the neck.

Risks: There is a low risk of radiation exposure.

After effects: There are no after effects.

Precautions: If you are nursing or there is any possibility of pregnancy, the doctor should be told in advance.

Bone Scan

This test is performed at an imaging center/hospital radiology center. The test itself usually takes about an hour; however, waiting time for the absorption of the tracer and between scans can be up to six hours.

Preparation: No x-rays using barium should be performed in the four days leading up to a bone scan. Fluid intake should be limited for four hours before the test. A hospital gown is worn, and jewelry and metal objects must be removed.

Risks: There is a low level of exposure to radiation. Reactions may include rash or swelling. Severe allergic reaction (anaphylaxis) is possible.

After effects: If occasional soreness or swelling occurs at the injection site, apply warm, moist compresses. If a rash develops or the swelling worsens, tell your doctor.

Precautions: If you are nursing or there is any possibility of pregnancy, tell your doctor in advance. The doctor should also be told about any allergies.

WHAT TO ASK YOUR DOCTOR ABOUT TESTS

While these are by no means all the questions that may occur to you, they will get you off to a good start.

What is the name of the test I am having?
Why do I need this test?
Your doctor's answer should include the full name of the test and whether the test is to diagnose disease or confirm a diagnosis, to help determine a course of treatment, or to eliminate certain medical possibilities or the possibility of other diseases.

Will I need other tests? Will you repeat this test?
How urgent is it that I have this test now?
Your doctor's answer should explain whether the results of this test may indicate that more tests will be needed, what those tests are, and why this test might need to be repeated. During the diagnostic process, the doctor will consider it important, if not urgent, to have you undergo tests that will help confirm your condition and plan a treatment.

What do I need to do to prepare for the test? What side effects or risks might there be? How long is the test likely to take?

The descriptions in this chapter are only a guide, as your doctor may have more detailed instructions or require a different selection of preparatory steps. Answers should, in general, be similar to the precautions and preparations outlined in this chapter.

How much does the test cost? Is it covered by insurance?

Your doctor may refer you to his office staff for information on cost and insurance coverage.

Where will the test be done, and what certifications are held by the facility doing the test?

The office staff may schedule the test for you and give you directions to the radiology center, if needed. The imaging center should be certified by the American Board of Radiology, which ensures that its staff is properly trained to handle equipment that is inspected and certified as safe. When you're discussing qualifications of doctors or technicians, listen for the words "board-certified" or "certified by the board" along with references to the American Medical Association, American College of Surgeons, or American Board of Radiology.

When will you get the results?
How will you communicate the results to me?

Your doctor will give you an estimate of how long it will take to get the test results. Your doctor is likely to suggest scheduling an appointment for you and your family to come in and discuss the results and their implications for you and your treatment plan. That's the ideal way to review the results. However, if you are more comfortable talking on the phone, then perhaps you might want to request a phone call instead.

Be cautious about asking questions if you aren't likely to understand the meaning of the answer. For example, if you ask, "Where did you do your residency?" the answer probably won't mean much to you unless you have some idea of which hospitals or universities provide high-quality training.

The key is to ask the questions that are important to you. If you want to know how you'll feel after a test, that's the question to ask. If you want to know whether you should eat a special diet or change your work habits, ask that.

WHAT TO TELL YOUR DOCTOR

When your doctor is considering a diagnosis of bladder cancer, what you do for a living and how you spend your time are important pieces of information. If your physician doesn't know where you've worked or what your job history is, make sure you talk about that as those facts may give him a clue as to why you developed bladder cancer.

If you have never mentioned that you started smoking again after quitting 15 years ago, now is the time to confess. It is clear that once bladder cancer has been diagnosed, continued smoking is an adverse outcome factor (i.e., the results of treatment are worse in people who continue to smoke).

If you have worries about little aches and pains, speak up. That occasional ache in the lower left abdomen might be an important signal of something to your doctor, even though you've convinced yourself that it only happens when you carry the garbage cans out to the curb on Tuesdays. If you've had a little burning when you urinate or notice a brownish discoloration sometimes, do tell the doctor.

Think about things that may have changed in your habits or your life. Do you have to take a nap every day, when just a year ago you were full of energy? Do you drink more water now? Or take three alcoholic drinks instead of one? Are your feet always cold? Do you take an herbal remedy, such as feverfew or black cohosh? Do you have much more indigestion or heartburn than you used to? Have you been losing weight?

You don't need to bombard your doctor with every detail of your life. Just make sure to mention your family history, changes in how you feel, what hurts, and the new symptoms you're having. ◆

Chapter 3

What the Tests Tell Your Doctor

WHEN THE TEST RESULTS ARRIVE

You've been through a battery of tests. A flexible cystoscopy. An IVP, a CT scan, perhaps even a surgical biopsy and bone scan. The diagnosis? You have bladder cancer.

Even though you may well have reason to be hopeful about your treatment and outlook, the words are serious and frightening. Most people diagnosed for the first time with bladder cancer have tumors that are limited to the bladder itself. In about 20 percent of first-time cases, the cancer will have spread deeply into the bladder wall or to surrounding tissue outside the bladder, and in roughly 3 percent of the first-time diagnoses, it will have spread to other organs and tissues in the body.

Bladder cancer isn't just one disease, however, and what type of cancer you have, how deeply it's embedded in the layers of the bladder, and whether it is superficial or invasive and has spread to other parts of the body are all important pieces of information to you and your doctor, not only to predict the progression of the disease, but also to determine what treatment is right for you.

Different types of cancer respond differently to different types of treatment, so it's important for your medical team to evaluate your test results carefully before deciding on a treatment plan.

What are doctors looking for when they evaluate your test results? They are looking for the *type* of cancer you have, the *appearance* and *shape* of the cancer cells, whether it is *superficial or invasive,* the *stage* of the cancer (how invasive the cancer is), the *grade* of the cancer (how abnormal the cancer cells appear under the microscope), and whether *multiple* types of tumors are present.

TYPES OF BLADDER CANCER

Bladder tumors are grouped into several types, according to the way the tumors appear under the microscope. Three common types of bladder cancer are:

- **Transitional cell cancer,** or TCC. Sometimes TCC is referred to as urothelial cancer. It can be localized on the surface or it may be invasive. (TCC will be discussed in more detail later in the chapter.)

  This is the most common type of bladder cancer, accounting for about 90 percent of all cases. In 2007, the American Cancer Society estimated that by the end of the year about 67,160 people would be diagnosed with bladder cancer – roughly 49,000 men and 18,000 women – and that of these diagnoses, cases of TCC would number about 60,450.

- **Squamous cell cancer.** This type accounts for about 5 percent to 10 percent of all bladder cancers and is usually an invasive cancer. Squamous means "resembling a scale" (which is flat and thin) or a scaly surface, and squamous cell cancer looks like skin cancer when viewed under a microscope. Among the causes of squamous cell development is the *schistosomiasis* parasite discussed in Chapter 1.

- **Adenocarcinoma.** This describes a tumor that is very similar in appearance to tumors of gland-forming cells in the intestinal tract. (*Adeno* means "gland.") It is often associated with the production of small amounts of mucus. Some adenocarcinomas occur in the urachus, a remnant of a fetal structure that connects the bladder to the umbilicus before birth. Adenocarcinomas, which are usually invasive, account for about 1 percent to 2 percent of bladder cancers.

In addition to the above types of bladder cancer, there are several extremely uncommon forms of the disease. One is **small cell anaplastic** bladder cancer. It is similar to small cell cancer, a rapidly growing cancer usually found in the lung, and shares a pattern of rapid growth and early spread to other parts of the body. It is not really clear why small cell tumors arise in the bladder, although it is thought that they start from neuro-endocrine cells. These small, dark, round cells found on the wall of the bladder and in other organs may play a part in the control of cellular growth.

Two quite rare forms of bladder cancer are bladder **sarcomas** and **choriocarcinoma**. Sarcomas are found in the muscle layers of the bladder. Choriocarcinoma is most often diagnosed among Asians in the Far East. Found in the bladder wall, it is an extremely rare tumor that seems to arise from small clusters of cells that paradoxically resemble part of the placenta.

Squamous cell, adenocarcinoma, and other rare forms of cancer are generally diagnosed and treated in much the same way as muscle-invasive bladder cancers, and their treatment will be discussed in Chapter 5.

TRANSITIONAL CELL CARCINOMA (TCC)

If you have been diagnosed with TCC, it can mean many different things. TCC is not a single type of cancer; it is classified by shape and whether it is restricted to the inner surface of the bladder (superficial to underlying tissues and muscle) or invasive, as well as by stage and grade of development.

The term "transitional cells" refers to how the cells appear under the microscope. Transitional cells share features with various types of cells normally found in the area of the bladder.

Your bladder is made up of several layers. On the innermost surface (which is next to where urine is stored) there is a layer of cells known as the transitional cell epithelium. It varies in thickness from three to seven cells.

If your doctor described your tumor as being confined to the transitional cell epithelium, it is a superficial tumor. About 70 percent to 80 percent of TCCs are noninvasive and superficial when diagnosed, although superficial tumors may eventually progress to a more invasive stage. One has to be careful using the term "superficial" as this does not necessarily mean that the tumor is safe and doesn't have a dangerous potential.

Invasive TCC means that the cancer has progressed into other layers of your bladder wall, such as the intermediate cell layer or the muscle.

SHAPES OF BLADDER CANCER

Your TCC will be classified as either papillary or flat in shape, although more than one kind of tumor may be present at the same time in the bladder.

Papillary tumors look like the fronds on a fern leaf or a bunch of tiny berries or grapes. Papillary tumors can be superficial or invasive. Most papillary tumors are malignant; however, the papilloma tumor is a relatively benign type of papillary TCC that typically is removed by surgery.

Other tumors appear to be flat and velvety and are more commonly called CIS, or carcinoma in situ. These tumors are only one cell in thickness.

STAGING AND GRADING OF BLADDER CANCER

Your doctor probably described your cancer stage in terms of letters and numerals, which you may not have understood.

Think of staging as a way of determining how deeply your cancer has penetrated into the bladder and muscle, surrounding tissue, or distant organs. The pathologist stages the tissue from your biopsy and your doctor uses that information along with your scan, cystoscopy, and x-ray results to determine where you are in the disease process and what treatment is best for you.

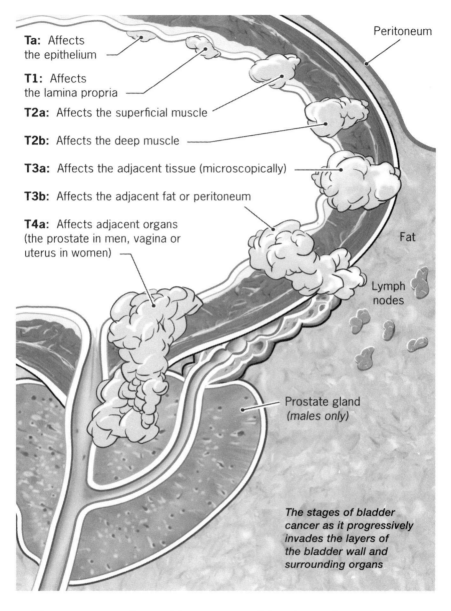

Ta: Affects the epithelium

T1: Affects the lamina propria

T2a: Affects the superficial muscle

T2b: Affects the deep muscle

T3a: Affects the adjacent tissue (microscopically)

T3b: Affects the adjacent fat or peritoneum

T4a: Affects adjacent organs (the prostate in men, vagina or uterus in women)

Peritoneum

Fat

Lymph nodes

Prostate gland (*males only*)

The stages of bladder cancer as it progressively invades the layers of the bladder wall and surrounding organs

If your test results – either scans or biopsies – show that cancer may have spread to other tissue or organs, your doctor will want to confirm that. Clarification of the stage of your cancer comes through looking at the cancer cells from those organs under the microscope. Tissue samples may be taken at the time of your biopsy, or sometimes a needle biopsy is done, bypassing the need for additional surgery.

Pathologists stage bladder-cancer tissue by using a standardized system known as TNM, which stands for tumor-nodes-metastases. A typical TNM might be T2aN1M0 (T-two-a-N-one-M-zero). Looks like mumbo-jumbo, doesn't it? Try thinking of it as medical short-hand, with each letter and numeral having a defined value that gives doctors and pathologists a specific, consistent way to describe how deeply a cancer has invaded the body's tissue and organs.

The TNM system uses the letters T, N, and M followed by numerals to describe the stage of invasiveness of your cancer.

The letter T followed by a numeral from 1 to 4 describes the depth of invasiveness of your tumor. The lower the number, the less invasive the cancer.

The T scale has additional, more detailed levels as well. These levels add the lowercase letters a and b to the T score to delineate more precisely how far into the bladder your cancer has spread and whether it has moved into other areas of your body. It fine-tunes the pathology information to better help your doctor make treatment recommendations.

The first T level refers to Ta or T1 tumors, which are superficial in nature. These noninvasive tumors can be papillary or CIS, and have penetrated only the epithelium or intermediate cell layers of the bladder. This is an early, highly treatable stage of bladder cancer. The Ta tumor is the least invasive (or most superficial) variant, whereas the T1 tumor shows the beginnings of invasion into the first layer of the bladder wall (before muscle is reached).

T2 tumors are invasive and have moved into the muscle layer of the bladder. The lower-case letters a and b are used to describe how far into the muscle the tumor has spread. A T2a tumor has not penetrated as deeply into the muscle as a T2b tumor.

T3 tumors, also further classified by the letters a and b, have penetrated beyond the bladder wall and into the fatty tissue surrounding the outside of the bladder. A T3a tumor is visible only with a microscope. A T3b tumor is visible in scans or to the naked eye during surgery.

A T4 tumor, the most serious and advanced of this local tumor grouping, has spread to other tissues or organs. A T4a tumor has invaded the nearby uterus or vagina in a woman or the prostate in a man. A T4b tumor has spread through the pelvic or abdominal wall into the body.

The letter N, followed by a numeral from 1 to 3, tells your doctor whether your cancer has spread to lymph nodes near the bladder and how deeply the cancer has penetrated the nodes. The higher the number, the more lymph nodes are involved and the more enlarged the nodes are.

The letter M followed by a 1 or a zero indicates whether your cancer has spread to lymph nodes in other parts of the body (beyond the pelvis) or to other organs such as the lungs or liver. A zero indicates that the cancer has not spread to other organs; the number 1 means that it has.

Once your doctor and pathologist have determined your TNM values, they will be combined and expressed as Roman numerals from zero to IV. Stage IV, for example, is the most advanced and serious stage of cancer. These stages help predict rates of survival five years after treatment; they range from 95 percent survival in the Stage 0 category to about 16 percent in the Stage IV category. The stage of your cancer also helps doctors decide how aggressive to be in recommending treatment options.

Once again, the terms Stage I or Stage IV are like medical shorthand, giving the physician a quick indication of overall prognosis and the general type of treatment that will be needed.

Grading the tumors is another tool for your doctor. Instead of measuring how invasive the tumor is, grading looks at how abnormal the tumor cells appear under the microscope. The more abnormal, or undifferentiated, the tumor cells are, the more likely it is your cancer will spread aggressively.

Pathologists use the numerals 1, 2, or 3 or the words low, medium, or high to describe how abnormal the tumor cells appear. A tumor graded either 3 or higher is the most likely to spread aggressively. In some systems, grading is done on a scale of 1 to 4.

CIS tumors, for example, are considered a high-grade bladder cancer because they characteristically have a high rate of progression to muscle-invasive tumors and also because they don't have any differentiated features. The paradox is that they are only one cell thick, which usually correlates with *lack* of invasion. About 50 percent of the people diagnosed with CIS who have no other types of tumor present in the bladder will eventually have the CIS invade the muscle.

WHAT DOES ALL THIS MEAN TO YOU?

While physicians and researchers can draw some general conclusions about bladder cancer and its diagnosis and treatment, it is not always easy to predict how it will behave.

Your physician and oncologist work with the pathologist to get an idea of your likely prognosis that is as accurate as possible, but the reality is that tumors of the same type don't always develop or progress in the same way. Nor do they always respond to treatment in the same way, and they don't always have a predictable pattern of recurrence.

For example, in general one can say that the more deeply into the bladder layers your cancer has spread, the more likely it is to recur. But sometimes superficial cancers become invasive. And sometimes they don't. Doctors and researchers don't yet have all the key indicators to predict which superficial cancers will become invasive and recur and which ones won't.

In general, if you've been diagnosed with superficial TCC, you can expect a 40 percent chance that the cancer won't recur, especially if you have a low-grade tumor where the cancer cells closely resemble normal bladder cells.

CARING4CANCER

Talk with your doctor about whether the publication *Caring4Cancer*, a magazine chock-full of information and articles of interest to cancer patients, their families, and caregivers, is right for you. Free copies of the publication are available in bulk only to doctors or health-care professionals at www.Caring4Cancer.com.

If you do have a recurrence of superficial TCC, there is a 60 percent chance that it will happen in the first year after treatment. And there is about a 25 percent chance that a recurrence will have progressed to a higher, more invasive, stage of the disease.

The stage, grade, and type of your cancer will strongly influence treatment options. (These will be discussed in the next two chapters.) They also are clues to whether your cancer might be aggressive, whether you might have a relapse or recurrence after treatment, and how hopeful the outlook is for a cure.

WHAT TO ASK YOUR DOCTOR ABOUT YOUR DIAGNOSIS

If your doctor tells you that you have bladder cancer, what you talk about next depends on the answers to these two questions.

What kind of bladder cancer do I have?

Expect your doctor to tell you whether your cancer is TCC, squamous cell, adenocarcinoma, or a rarer form of cancer and to give you a general explanation of how the type of cancer you have generally behaves, including whether your type of cancer often recurs, metastasizes, or is considered highly treatable.

What stage and grade is my tumor, and what does that mean?

Your doctor is likely to categorize your cancer with a letter, numeral, and stage – perhaps something like T2aN1M0 Stage I – and will explain what those symbols mean by describing how deeply the cancer has invaded your body, how abnormal the tumor cells are, and whether the cancer has spread.

When you are comfortable with the answers to the above questions, you'll be ready to move on and talk about treatment options. This is a good time to talk with your doctor about your treatment team. You'll want to know who will be on it, what part each doctor will play in your care, who will talk with you about your treatment plan, and who will serve as your "contact point" for questions or concerns.

TO HELP YOU TALK ABOUT CANCER

- **The National Cancer Institute** offers articles such as "What It's Like for You" and "Taking Time: Support for People with Cancer" at its website (www.cancer.gov). You can also call 1-800-422-6237 (1-800-4-CANCER) to find out about available publications and brochures.

- **Cleveland Clinic** offers a brochure titled "What to Say to Children About Cancer" that you can download at http://cms.clevelandclinic.org/cancer/documents/kidscancer.pdf. For information about cancer support groups at Cleveland Clinic, call the Cancer Answer Line at 1-800-862-7798.

- **The American Cancer Society** offers a number of articles on coping with cancer, including "Helping Children When a Family Member Has Cancer" and "Talking with Children About Cancer" at www.cancer.org. You can also call 1-800-227-2345 (1-800-ACS-2345) for information on ordering.

- **The Cancer Survivors Network** is a forum or message board at the American Cancer Society website (www.cancer.org) where people can ask questions and share information and resources with others dealing with cancer.

- **Your hospital's social work department** will have counseling and resources available for you and your family. Just ask your doctor to put you in touch with the appropriate office.

FIRST STEPS IN TALKING WITH YOUR FAMILY ABOUT CANCER

You'll also be talking to family members about your diagnosis and treatment plans. Here are some pointers to keep in mind.

- Let your family, especially children or grandchildren, know what's happening. Children, even very young children, pick up on worry and anxiety, and easily imagine the worst if information is kept secret.
- To the extent that you are comfortable doing so, share your feelings, and encourage your loved ones to share theirs.
- Do take advantage of available resources. There are excellent websites and books available about coping with cancer. (See the section on Resources at the back of this book for an extensive list.) You can also ask your doctor to refer you to a social worker or support group.
- When possible, couch discussions in hopeful and reassuring words by telling your loved ones that you feel positive about your treatment.
- When talking about cancer with children, keep information age-appropriate. The National Cancer Institute has a guide called *Tips for Talking With Children of Different Ages* that you can obtain at www.cancer.gov.
- With your family members, agree to give each other permission to feel stressed or worried or angry – or even happy – without feeling guilty.
- Acknowledge that there may be tough times, but recognize that caring and love will help get you through them.
- Acknowledge that things will change. Talk about changes as they occur.
- Talk often with family and loved ones. Speak from your hearts.
- Expect lots of questions. Expect some disagreements. Expect times when you wish that things could go back to the way they were before you had cancer. And expect deeply loving moments with the people you love most.

DIAGNOSIS CASE STUDY: DIANE, AGE 56

Diane knew something was wrong when her family doctor left a message on her voice mail to call about her test results. Usually after her annual physical she'd receive a letter that said "Everything's fine, see you next year."

By the time she got through to Dr. W, her stomach was churning with worry.

"Diane, your urinalysis showed some microscopic blood in your urine. It's something I think we should check out. Have you noticed any visible blood in your urine or had any changes in urine function? Do you feel that you have to go more often? Do you have any pain when urinating?"

Only the previous day Diane's husband had complained that she couldn't shop for more than 10 minutes without heading for a bathroom. But she wasn't having any pain or visible blood. That was good, wasn't it?

Dr. W agreed that it was a good sign. Still, Diane should see a urologist.

"It may be nothing more than bladder irritation from the analgesic you take for your arthritis, Diane. But because of your increased urge to urinate, I want to err on the side of caution. Let me switch you to the appointment desk."

At the Urologist's Office

Diane didn't expect Dr. H, the urologist, to do much more than talk on her first visit. So she was surprised when her doctor, after asking Diane a number of questions, including whether she ever smoked and what she did for a living, said that she wanted to perform a flexible cystoscopy. Even though the doctor explained the procedure and assured her that she'd feel fine afterward, Diane was glad that her husband, Carl, had driven her to her appointment.

The flexible cystoscopy wasn't as unpleasant as it sounded, although Diane was uncomfortable when the doctor filled her bladder with fluid and asked her to hold it in.

A few minutes into the procedure, she said, "I'm going to snip some tissue, Diane. You shouldn't feel anything except some minor discomfort. There is an abnormal growth in the upper right quadrant that I think we should biopsy."

After the cystoscopy, which was over in less than 10 minutes, Diane hurried to the bathroom to void the liquid she'd been holding for what seemed like hours and then met Carl in the doctor's office. When she mentioned that there had been a little blood in her urine, Dr. H assured her that that was normal after a biopsy.

"As I told you, Diane, there is tissue with an abnormal appearance in your bladder, which means that there is a significant probability that the growth is cancer. However, we won't know for sure until we get the biopsy results. That will take about a week. In the meantime, I'd like you to have a couple other tests so that we have a thorough picture of what's going on with you."

Diane gasped. Even though she'd been expecting bad news ever since the doctor had told her during the cystoscopy that there was a growth present, the word cancer hit her like a sucker punch.

"Are you sure it's cancer?"

"As sure as I can be without seeing the actual biopsy results, Diane. What I'm not sure about right now is what stage the cancer is or whether it may have spread, and that's what these other tests, along with the biopsy, will help us determine."

Both Carl and Diane were stunned. Diane had been feeling fine, and until some lab tech had found a few drops of blood in her urine a week ago, she'd thought her health was great. And now, in the space of a few days, she was being told she had cancer. It was hard to process.

Carl said, "Is bladder cancer ... a bad kind of cancer? I mean, some types are pretty treatable."

"It really depends on the biopsy results, Carl. There are different types of bladder cancer, some very treatable and some very aggressive. Sometimes we catch it very early, yet the outcome is not what we'd like. We just don't have enough information yet to know in Diane's case."

The urologist asked questions about Diane's weight and energy level. Was she having any new or persistent aches and pains?

Diane replied that she was fine, no problems, but Carl reminded her that she had complained recently about a pain in her abdomen.

Diane could tell that Carl's comment concerned the doctor.

"What are you thinking? That maybe the cancer has spread?" Diane was afraid of the answer, but she asked anyway.

"I don't know what it means right now, Diane. It could be nothing more than gas in your abdomen. Let's get the tests going and take a look at the results before we start jumping to conclusions." Dr. H tapped her pen on the folder and said, "I'm going to write orders for a chest x-ray, some more blood work, and a CT scan."

After explaining the test procedures, she gave Diane brochures on bladder cancer.

"I know this is all pretty overwhelming right now," she said. "I encourage you to think about what we've discussed today. Read the brochures I gave you and start a list of questions. When we've got all the information from the tests, we'll sit down and go over it together in detail. I'm going to have Nancy make your test appointments for you before you leave and schedule another appointment with me a week after your last test."

"That long? I'll go crazy," said Diane. "Can't we hurry it up?"

"It's hard to wait, I know, but I need time to get the reports back and look them over. In the meantime, try not to worry. Keep in mind that you're 56 and that overall your health is good. These are very positive things working in your favor."

Dr. H stood up and said, "Call my office any time you have questions. I can't always stop and talk to you right then, but I'm very good about returning phone calls. And don't think your questions are dumb – if you're worried about something, even if it's something minor, I want to know. Okay?"

Within minutes, Nancy had set up all the appointments and handed Diane pre-printed sheets with instructions on what to eat and what to avoid before the tests.

During the ride home, Diane felt as if she were looking at different scenery in a different world. On one hand, everything seemed the same, but sharper. Crisper. The air was cold and fresh, the sky more blue than it had been on the ride to the urologist's office. Yet she also felt focused inward, slightly removed from everything that was happening around her. It took an effort to speak, to listen to and understand what she was hearing, as if all her energy were being pulled into a fragile center from which the word *cancer, cancer, cancer* was drumming through her head. Even though Carl was sitting right beside her, Diane felt very alone.

Over the next two weeks, Diane joked to Carl that she was taking her clothes off and putting them back on so many times that she was tempted just to wear her bathrobe to future appointments so that she wouldn't have to bother with buttons and zippers. The only test that bothered her was the CAT scan; she reacted to the solution they had injected into her vein and itched like crazy for the next few days, but this quieted down quickly when she contacted the doctor, who gave her some anti-allergy medicine.

Diane realized that whatever the diagnosis turned out to be, it wouldn't be just her diagnosis. It would be Carl's and the girls', too.

With each test, Diane became more worried. *If I could just forget about all this for a few hours and get some sleep,* she thought, *it would be easier.* Carl wanted to tell their daughters what was happening, but Diane flatly refused.

"Carl, it's hard enough to keep myself from flying to pieces over this, and you … well, sometimes you look at me as if I'm about to dissolve in front of your eyes. The girls have their families to take care of, and they'd be so upset. Just wait until we know what we're facing. Please? I don't want to worry them any more than is necessary."

Carl agreed, but she still caught him looking at her with a sad, frightened look. She realized that whatever the diagnosis turned out to be, it wouldn't be just *her* diagnosis. It would be Carl's and the girls', too.

Telling the Family

About the time Max was talking with his physician and learning about his treatment options (see Chapter 1), Diane and Carl were sitting down to an early dinner with their three adult daughters and their husbands.

Diane still felt shell-shocked from the test and biopsy results. She and Carl had decided to tell all three girls about what was happening at the same time, when they were all together. The girls knew something was up, though. It was unheard of for Diane to invite the adults to dinner without the grandchildren.

After dinner, Carl poured coffee for everyone. Diane took a deep breath and said, "Dad and I have something to tell you."

Despite her best intentions, her tears started to flow. Carl took over.

"Mom has been diagnosed with bladder cancer," he said, holding Diane's hand. "It's a kind of cancer called 'invasive cancer,' and it's not a good kind of cancer to have. It's what the doctors call high grade, and it's pretty advanced."

"How advanced?" asked Neil, a pharmacist.

"It's Stage III," Diane said. Then, with a weak grin, she added, "You probably want the details. It's a T3aN1M0 tumor."

Neil nodded, and Carl went on. "But … the doc thinks there's a good chance that surgery and chemo treatments will knock the cancer for a loop and give Mom a fighting chance to beat this."

"What about metastasis? Has it spread?" said Neil.

Diane's voice shook with sobs. "It hasn't spread to any distant point, but it has extended locally, beyond the bladder."

"Oh my God, Mom," Becka, Neil's wife, said. "That's … that's unbelievable. You're fine. You cooked dinner. How did this happen? When did you find out?"

"I had a physical a month ago, and there was blood in my urine," said Diane. "I didn't see it – the lab found it. And it just went from there. A biopsy. A CAT scan. A chest x-ray. Lots of tests, and lots of worry and waiting."

"I wish you had told us, Mom. We could have worried with you," said Donna, the oldest. Her voice was chilly.

"Well, Dad and I didn't want to sound the alarm unnecessarily. We wanted some answers before we talked to you girls. And, now we have some answers. It's cancer. I'm going to start chemo the day after tomorrow, and then I'll go in for surgery in a couple months. I know I'm going to need you girls to help out. I don't know how bad I'll feel, but at least after the surgery, I'm going to need a hand cooking for your Dad and cleaning this house."

A chorus of "We'll help, of course we will," accompanied a round of sniffles and sobs. Carl reached for the box of tissues he'd put on the end table right before dinner. "Here. I figured you girls would need these. You always have been criers, the whole bunch of you."

Gail, the youngest, laughed shakily. "Yeah, that's us, the sob sisters." She blew her nose. "What's the surgery all about? To remove the tumor?"

Diane shook her head. "No, it's to remove my bladder. Which is not an appealing idea, but the surgeon said that chances are good they can make me an artificial bladder out of my intestine and connect it so that I can go to the bathroom normally. If that doesn't work, then it might have to be a little more complicated, with a drain or something. But girls, that's the least of it if I'm healthy afterward, right?"

Gail couldn't imagine her mother, who cared so much about how she looked and what she wore and who always looked fashionably chic, having to deal with emptying a urine bag, internal or external. The whole thing felt sad and ... wrong.

"Mom, I'm really scared for you. Are you scared?" Gail asked.

Diane nodded and then said, "No, that's not true. I'm not really scared. I'm sad that I might have fewer years to be on this earth than I expected. I'm sad that Dad might be alone, and I'm sad that I might not see the grandkids grow up and that I'll miss good things in your lives. But I'm not scared."

Donna had been getting angry as the conversation went on. Why did they try to do it all alone? Dad driving all the way downtown by himself to take Mom to tests. They're so stubborn sometimes – and who has to pick up the pieces? Us. Me and Becka and Gail, just like when Dad insisted on taking down the screens himself and fell off the ladder. Who mowed the lawn and took the trash out for weeks?

Finally Donna's feelings erupted. "I can't believe you couldn't trust us enough to tell us before, Mom. I mean, it's kind of a lot to dump on us all at once, you know. Cancer. Surgery. Chemotherapy. At least you could have let us know that you were having tests. How did you think we'd react, Mom?"

Diane was shocked by her daughter's anger. But then, the social worker had told them that people react differently to deeply emotional news. Some cry, some withdraw, some experience anger or paralyzing fear. Even so, she hadn't expected any of the girls to lash out. In a small way, she resented Donna's outburst. *I'm the one with cancer,* she thought. *I'm the one who's facing the possibility of wearing a urinary pouch and feeling miserable from chemo. I'm the one who might die. Why should I have to worry about soothing Donna's feelings? She should be worrying about ME, not turning everything around to make this be about her.*

As if she'd read her mother's mind, Donna came over and knelt by Diane's chair. "I'm sorry, Mom, I'm just … freaked. I love you, and I can't stand the thought of you hurting or …"

"Dying." Diane said it for her. Donna nodded.

"Hey, don't give up on me so easily. I have every reason to believe that the treatments will cure me. My doctor said I have a 50-50 chance of a cure, and even if the cancer can't be cured, she's confident that treatment will buy me a remission with a good amount of time. I'm going to try not to think the worst, but if it comes to that, we'll deal with it, honey. And I promise that I won't hold back information anymore."

Carl cleared his throat. "Let's keep in mind that Mom's really going to need us for a while, okay? And," he said in a dramatic voice, "we have something else to talk about."

Gail groaned. "I can't take much more tonight, Dad."

"It's about Thanksgiving," said Diane. "Someone else is going to have to cook the turkey this year." ◆

Chapter 4

Early Stage Bladder Cancer

When applied to TCC, the term "superficial" can be misleading, and some doctors would like to see the term discontinued. Many people equate the term "superficial" with "not very risky," which isn't always the case.

In general, superficial TCC at the low or intermediate risk levels is a highly treatable form of bladder cancer with a good chance for an excellent outcome despite a moderate to high rate of recurrence (depending on the extent and nature of the tumor). But as we discussed in Chapter 3, some superficial TCCs are considered high risk and carry an elevated chance that the cancer will not only recur, but may have progressed to a more dangerous stage when it does recur.

Luckily, only about 20 percent of those who experience a recurrence are diagnosed with a more advanced type of bladder cancer. What this means is that "superficial" bladder cancer, if and when if recurs, will usually come back again as a superficial cancer that can be managed by local means. However, understanding your prognosis and being informed about the cancer's possibility of recurrence are important parts of your overall treatment process.

Make sure that your multidisciplinary team – which may include your urologist, oncologist, pathologist, and radiation oncologist – welcomes your active involvement in your treatment plan and thoroughly explains each step of the process to you. It is worth mentioning that noninvasive bladder cancer is usually managed by a urologist with support from the pathologist and usually does not require a full multidisciplinary team unless it recurs repeatedly.

Your treatment plan for superficial TCC will include some or all of the following: resection, intravesical chemotherapy, and immunotherapy, which this chapter will discuss in detail, and less frequently cystectomy and perhaps even prostatectomy, which are discussed in Chapter 5.

The following descriptions are of a general nature; your experience during your actual medical procedure may differ from what is discussed here.

BIOPSY AND RESECTION

Most likely at this point you've undergone some of the diagnostic tests discussed in Chapter 2. You've had tissue biopsied and classified as superficial TCC, and you probably underwent a flexible cystoscopy, during which your doctor thoroughly examined your bladder wall and made a "map" of the location of abnormal tissue or tumors that other diagnostic tests have confirmed. Sometimes more than one tumor will be present in the bladder, so your urologist will be very careful to look at the whole organ from the inside.

The next step for you is likely to be resection (removal of the tumor), unless you've already had a surgical biopsy or rigid cystoscopy. In that case, your doctor may have done a resection to avoid your having to undergo a second surgical procedure under anesthesia.

Undergoing a resection sounds more intimidating than it actually is. Think of it as the removal of the piece of the bladder where the tumor or abnormal cells are growing. This may effectively clear the bladder of tumor, bringing it to a state where only healthy tissue remains.

When you have a bladder resection by means of a cystoscopy, as opposed to invasive surgery, you won't have an incision or stitches, as no external cutting or incision is required.

Resecting (sometimes called endoscopic resection) is performed under general anesthesia in a hospital setting. Your doctor will use a resectoscope, which resembles a somewhat larger cystoscope. Like a cystoscope, it has a lighted lens and is introduced into your bladder through your urethra. (Don't worry; you'll be asleep under anesthesia and receiving pain medication while this is happening.)

Your doctor will fill your bladder with water or a nonirritating clear liquid such as glycine, which expands the bladder walls and makes it easier to see tumors and abnormalities. Guided by the map made during the initial cystoscopy, your doctor will use a small wire loop (through which a high-energy electrical current runs) to remove the cancer, a margin of healthy tissue, and a small amount of muscle. Any remaining cells are removed with an electric current or sometimes a high-powered laser. Sometimes your doctor will also take a few random tissue samples from other areas of your bladder to make sure that abnormal cells aren't developing elsewhere. The tumor, healthy tissue, and muscle are then sent to your pathologist for examination.

A small amount of muscle tissue is included in the tissue sample so that the pathologist can make sure the tumor hasn't spread into the muscle wall. A margin of healthy tissue is taken to help decrease the chances that abnormal cells remain in the bladder.

Resection is usually carried out as outpatient surgery. This means that you probably will be able to go home the same day. (You'll need to bring a driver with you as you'll still be recovering from anesthesia and won't be sufficiently alert to drive a car.) You may have some blood in your urine for a few days after a resection, and you may experience pain or stinging upon urination. The stinging urination can be eased by drinking lots of fluids and by taking simple pain medications prescribed by your urologist. If either condition lingers longer than two or three days, if other painful conditions occur, or if the bleeding becomes extensive, call your doctor right away.

In some circumstances, your doctor may choose to insert a catheter into your bladder for a short time (usually only one to two days) after the surgery, to prevent blood clots from obstructing the flow of urine and causing discomfort. The catheter allows blood and urine to gently drain out of the bladder and also allows your doctor to irrigate your bladder to promote complete healing of the resected area.

On rare occasions, doctors will recommend another resection procedure. Sometimes the pathologist wants to biopsy muscle tissue from deeper in the bladder wall. And sometimes the tumor is too large to be safely removed all at once.

Sometimes, in an alternative procedure, lasers (high-energy light beams) are used to remove superficial TCC tumors. While this is slightly more comfortable than resection for you as a patient, the laser often destroys the tumor tissue, leaving nothing for pathologists to examine. The lack of pathology may limit your medical team's ability to predict recurrence and target your follow-up plan.

If you have been diagnosed with a low-risk tumor, resection may be the only treatment recommended by your medical team. Or your team may recommend a course of intravesical therapy, too.

INTRAVESICAL THERAPY

Intravesical is a medical term meaning "within the bladder." Intravesical therapy, therefore, means that treatment – in this case a solution containing anti-cancer drugs – is placed directly in the bladder instead of being given to you as a pill to swallow or as an injection.

The treatment is given as a liquid poured through an ordinary urinary catheter, the same device that is usually used to drain urine from the bladder. In this case, the flow of fluid is reversed, with the medication being injected gently up through the catheter into the inside of the bladder. Think of it this way: Remember when you were a kid and filled balloons with water? If you imagine the bladder as that balloon, filled not with water but with liquid medication sloshing around inside, you'll have a good idea of how intravesical therapy works.

Intravesical therapy has been used for about 30 years as a preventive treatment to reduce the recurrence rate for superficial bladder cancer. It is believed that intravesical therapy works because it destroys cancer cells that may remain "floating" in the bladder after resection, thereby reducing the possibility of a recurrence. It also may be absorbed directly into any remaining tumor tissue, causing destruction of the tumor.

There are two types of intravesical therapy, **chemotherapy** and **immunotherapy,** with numerous treatment options within each therapy group.

During intravesical therapy, a solution of anti-cancer drugs is inserted into the bladder through a catheter.

Your medical team will take a number of things into consideration when deciding which intravesical treatment option is best for you. Their goal is to balance the effectiveness of the treatment with possible side effects and long-term risks based on the type and seriousness of your cancer.

Aggressive treatment options with possibly serious side effects may well be the right choice if you're dealing with a type of cancer that has a high recurrence rate and often comes back in a more life-threatening form. On the other hand, if your cancer is low risk and has a lesser chance of recurring, a more conservative approach might be taken.

Regardless of whether you're advised to take chemotherapy or immunotherapy, both are administered the same way. The procedure can be performed either at the hospital about one to seven days after your resection or in your doctor's office if a series of weekly treatments is recommended. The timing depends somewhat on how extensive the resection has been.

First your doctor will numb your urethra with a topical gel and insert a disposable catheter, which will be used to fill the bladder with the solution. The catheter is removed after your bladder is full, and you'll be asked to concentrate on not passing urine for a time, holding the solution inside while you get up and move around. Walking, sitting, and standing while the solution is held in your bladder causes it to slosh around and completely coat inside the bladder walls. After an hour or so, you'll void the solution just as you would pass urine. In most cases, you'll be asked to minimize your fluid intake before the procedure so that your bladder won't also be filling with urine that will put additional pressure on your bladder.

The **chemotherapy** drugs that are used in this way include doxorubicin (brand name Adriamycin), epirubicin (Pharmorubicin), mitomycin C (Mutamycin), and occasionally thiotepa (Thioplex). Chemotherapy solutions have proved effective in reducing recurrence rates by about 30 percent. However, chemotherapy has little or no effect in preventing superficial cancer from progressing to a more serious stage. What this means is that chemotherapy will often stop the superficial cancer from coming back; however, studies have shown that if the cancer should come back, chemotherapy will not prevent it from coming back in a deeper or more aggressive form. For this reason, the urologist will follow you carefully to ensure that you are not caught unawares by a worsening tumor.

Side effects are fewer from intravesical chemotherapy than from chemotherapy by injection, since a smaller proportion of the chemotherapy drugs gets into the bloodstream during intravesical therapy. Therefore side effects are more likely to be limited to the bladder itself, such as the feeling of having a very nasty bladder infection, rather than affecting the whole body.

Side effects that you might have after intravesical chemotherapy include skin irritation or rash, cystitis (inflammation or irritation of the bladder), leaking of fluid, allergic reaction, and in some infrequent cases a narrowing of the ureters or urethra, making it difficult to urinate.

Less commonly there are some "whole body" side effects, such as interference with bone-marrow production (myelosuppression), if the chemotherapy agent is absorbed through the bladder. This usually happens only if intravesical chemotherapy is used soon after resection of an extensive primary bladder cancer, leaving behind a temporarily damaged surface that has blood vessels that can take up the drugs.

Immunotherapy means the use of medicines that stimulate the immunity of your own body (i.e., your immune system) to attack your cancer through the immune response.

Intravesical **immunotherapy** has been used since 1976. Immunotherapy means the use of medicines that stimulate the immunity of your own body (i.e., your immune system) to attack your cancer through the immune response. It's effective in reducing recurrences and in preventing recurrent cancer from progressing to a more serious stage in both superficial TCC and CIS.

A bacterium (a germ or microbe) called Bacille Calmette Guérin (BCG) is commonly used for intravesical immunotherapy. This is actually the germ that causes a type of tuberculosis, but it is used in a very weakened or modified form that usually doesn't present any

BCG TREATMENTS

BCG is a live bacterial strain in the tuberculosis family. While it has been modified so that there is little chance of your contracting TB from the bacteria, care needs to be taken while you're receiving BCG treatments. If you're a man, for about six hours after receiving a treatment you should sit down to urinate to avoid splashing urine outside the toilet. About six hours following a treatment both men and women should pour a cup of full-strength bleach into the toilet before flushing. Make sure to wash your hands thoroughly. If urine splashes outside the toilet, wipe it up with a cloth dipped in bleach water and thoroughly wash the cloth (and any clothing that may have been splashed) in hot water.

danger at all. BCG works by attracting immune-system cells to the bladder and activating them (turning them "on") to affect the cancer cells present.

Although BCG is highly effective, it also has some toxic side effects, and as such is used primarily as a treatment for patients with high-risk types of superficial bladder cancer and those who have had repeated recurrences or CIS.

Side effects may include a burning sensation in the bladder as well as fatigue, chills, and fever. A prolonged high fever and general feeling of being ill may be a sign that the BCG bacteria have spread through the body. Because BCG is the bacterium that causes a type of tuberculosis, antibiotics used to treat tuberculosis are usually prescribed when an infection occurs shortly after BCG immunotherapy.

Another type of immunotherapy is interferon. This is naturally produced in your body's cells and works much as BCG does in stimulating your body to attack cancer cells in the bladder. Temporary side effects, which usually disappear once interferon therapy is stopped, include muscle and bone aches, fatigue, vomiting, and headaches.

HOW MUCH? HOW OFTEN?

In almost all cases, intravesical therapy (chemotherapy or immunotherapy) is most effective when the first dose is given 6 to 24 hours after resection. Sometimes a single dose is given as a prophylactic (preventative) measure and is not repeated. More commonly, you'll have one dose immediately after resection and then five more treatments on a weekly basis in your doctor's office. In some cases, if a large tumor has been resected, leaving a larger area of ulcerated bladder surface, intravesical chemotherapy will be delayed for a few days to prevent the drug's being absorbed through the damaged surface lining of the bladder. Your doctor may recommend a follow-up cystoscopy after the intravesical treatments are completed.

Keep in mind that there are several types of superficial bladder cancer, some of which have a high risk of recurrence or progression to a more serious stage. Treatment options, including resection and intravesical therapy, are different for each person and depend upon each person's circumstances.

For example, you may start talking to someone in your urologist's waiting room who has had great results and few side effects from a single dose of mitomycin C (MCC) chemotherapy. Even more impressive, he hasn't had a recurrence since his diagnosis three years ago.

You, on the other hand, are on your fourth BCG treatment, and each one leaves you feeling as if you have severe bladder irritation for several days afterwards. "No side effects and no recurrences" sounds like a better deal than what you're experiencing. So why wasn't MCC prescribed for you?

There could be many reasons. Maybe you have a type of cancer that is high risk or that responds well to BCG. What you don't want to do is become overwhelmed with worry about whether you're getting the right therapy or whether your doctor is treating your disease properly. Talk to your urologist. Understand your treatment and why it was recommended for you. Having confidence in your treatment plan is very important. Don't wonder about these things. Ask questions!

OTHER TREATMENTS

On rare occasions, even with a diagnosis of superficial TCC, part or all of the bladder needs to be removed. If your doctor feels that cystectomy or partial cystectomy (removal of part of the bladder) is called for, he'll discuss the reasons with you and explain why this approach is preferable to any alternative, less radical treatments that may exist. (See Chapter 5 for a discussion of cystectomy.)

WHAT HAPPENS NEXT?

Apart from giving up smoking, follow-up is the best preventive measure there is for bladder cancer.

For the first two years after treatment, you'll have a cystoscopy, usually every three to four months. If no further tumors are found during that time, follow-up every six months for an additional two years is usually adequate, with annual cystoscopies after that. Since bladder cancer can recur in later years, most doctors in the United States prefer to do annual follow-up cystoscopies for the rest of the patient's life. Some physicians will reduce the number of cystoscopies by alternating them with the urine cytology test (discussed in Chapter 2), whereby urine is collected and examined for the presence of cancer cells under a microscope.

PREVENTION

First and foremost, don't smoke. Don't ride in a car with a smoker. If possible, don't live in a house with a smoker – or at least try to make sure that all smoking occurs outdoors. Become an advocate for living in a smoke-free environment.

Apart from avoiding known carcinogens (cancer-causing substances) and advocating for a general reduction in the use of products known to cause cancer, there is little one can do to prevent a recurrence of bladder cancer.

There is some discussion in the medical community about whether routine screening for blood in the urine might lead to earlier diagnosis for those who are at high risk of recurrence. At present, these screening tests are not accurate enough to be completely reliable, but as technology advances, so will the sophistication of such tests, enabling people like you to monitor their disease more frequently and with far more comfort.

Many people claim that diet, antioxidants, and various other healthful lifestyle approaches are helpful in the battle against cancer or in retarding the progress of cancer. Frankly, the data are pretty thin, but we believe that it is a good idea to take regular exercise and consume a "heart-healthy" diet low in cholesterol and fats and high in whole grains, legumes, fruits, and vegetables. This doesn't apply only to the battle against cancer; it just makes good sense when you're trying to live a long and healthy life. In light of some of the published medical data, it is probably also a good idea to keep your fluid consumption up, as there is some evidence that bladder cancers occur less frequently in people who have high fluid intake.

WHAT IF THE CANCER COMES BACK?

What happens if your cancer comes back? Most likely, your medical team has prepared you for the possibility. The signature of bladder cancer is that it can and often does come back, most often in the first two years.

If it does come back, most of the time it's treated just as it was when the tumor was originally diagnosed. You'll go through the same battery of tests or something similar, and the same grading and staging process. And you'll probably have the same treatment options, although hopefully, as medicine advances, you'll have more and better treatment options available. Of course, if the cancer is more advanced than it was the first time, some differences in treatment will be required. (See Chapter 5 for details.)

The key to managing bladder cancer is to tell your doctor promptly if you experience blood in your urine or any of the other symptoms discussed in Chapter 1. (Remember, blood in the urine doesn't always signal cancer. It might be there only because of infection.) The earlier a recurrence is found, the better your chances for a good outcome. Don't wait until your next appointment or decide that you'll mention it in six weeks when you're due for your annual cystoscopy. Call your doctor now.

WHAT TO ASK YOUR DOCTOR ABOUT TREATMENTS

These questions will help you get a clear sense of what happens next. As always, they are only a starting point. Anything else that occurs to you is a worthy question and should be addressed.

What can I expect after surgery? What are the risks of resection?

You may have a catheter in your urethra to help prevent bleeding or blockages. In that case, you may have to stay in the hospital for a day or two following surgery. (When possible, resection is performed on an outpatient basis.) If you are released the same day, your doctor should review possible after effects such as frequent urination, urine blockage, bladder infection, or blood in the urine and let you know what you should do if you experience any of them. Make sure you ask whether there are any restrictions on activity or exercise.

Your doctor also should explain any risks, such as blood clots or perforation of the bladder.

What if I have to have intravesical chemotherapy?

It is likely that your urologist will be the one to administer intravesical chemotherapy, although occasionally you will be referred to a medical oncologist for this. The physician who gives this treatment can give you details about when you will receive the chemotherapy (before or after surgery), how long the course of treatment will be, what side effects you might have (such as bladder irritation or discomfort), and what risks are involved. Make sure you know which members of your team you can speak with if you have questions or concerns about your chemotherapy or about symptoms and side effects of treatment. Your doctor should tell you when to be concerned about side effects and what to do about them (e.g., make an office appointment or go to the emergency room).

What if immunotherapy is prescribed?

There are numerous commercial brands of preparations used for immunotherapy and numerous treatment plans for administering them. You'll want to know the details of the immunotherapy plan for you as well as what specific side effects (such as burning or chills and fatigue) are associated with the immunotherapy preparation you receive. Your doctor should tell you which members of your medical team to speak with if you experience ongoing problems or have concerns. Your doctor should tell you when to be concerned about side effects and what to do (e.g., make an office appointment or go to the emergency room).

When should I come back for a checkup and what can I do to prevent a recurrence? What about screening tests for a recurrence?

Make sure that your doctor schedules a follow-up cystoscopy in about three months and discusses whether any of the newer screening tests for bladder-cancer "markers" might be appropriate for you. If you are still smoking, your doctor should encourage you to enroll in a program to help you quit. Make sure that your doctor reviews the symptoms that might signal a recurrence and discusses what you should do if you experience any of them.

What about having sex? Drinking alcohol? Can I continue to take vitamins or should I stop? How long will I have to be off work? Can I drive?

Feel free to ask these types of lifestyle questions as well as any others that concern your personal hobbies or activities. For example, if you love to golf, ask when you can tee off again. If you babysit your grandchildren twice a week, ask when you're likely to feel up to doing so. Do you have a vacation to Maui planned for next month? Make sure you ask whether there's any reason you won't be able to go.

TREATMENT CASE STUDY: MAX

Max told everyone that his resection surgery was "a piece of cake." Jean rolled her eyes when she heard him say that and added, "A piece of cake for him, maybe, but he drove the nurses crazy with his jokes."

Humor was Max's way of dealing with the worry and stress. It kept him from thinking about the word "cancer."

He couldn't slough off the worry, though, when his son-in-law started bringing over stacks of information he'd copied from the Internet about treatment for bladder cancer.

"Dad, I know you have a lot of faith in this doctor, but the treatment he's giving you, this BCG, is powerful stuff. I mean, if you splash urine with live BCG on the toilet seat, Mom could pick up the bacteria. She could get TB. So could you. Did this doctor even suggest anything else? Like mitomycin C, for example?"

Max shook his head. "No, he said this BCG was the best for the kind of cancer I have. That's good enough for me, Don. So I test positive for TB for the next few years? At least I'm not radioactive, right?"

Max knew that his son-in-law meant well, but all the talk about other treatments was starting to upset Jean.

On the way to Max's next appointment with Dr. P, Jean pulled out a wad of the printouts from her purse and said, "Just ask him about some of this information, okay? Please? I just want to make sure you're getting the right care."

"Fine." Max muttered all the way into the office and was still mumbling about the "stupid Internet" when the doctor came in.

"How are things? Ready to get started next week?" Dr. P glanced at the papers in Jean's hand and knew what was coming. He'd had plenty of patients do research on the Internet and in fact encouraged them to do so, as long as they were using reputable websites.

"You've been researching," said Dr. P. "Do you have any questions?"

Jean spoke up and explained their son-in-law's concern about BCG. She handed Dr. P the sheaf of articles. He flipped through them and pulled a couple out.

"First of all, let's talk about website information. Some of what you've brought with you comes from good sites that have solid medicine, such as the People Living With Cancer and the chemocare.com websites. But these," he waved the articles he'd pulled from the pile, "these are from websites that don't update their information and don't have it reviewed by medical experts."

He gave them a checklist and told them how to determine whether the websites were reputable.

"What about getting TB? That really worries me and seems to be what upsets my son-in-law, too," said Jean.

Dr. P explained that BCG is a live strain of the bacteria that causes TB, but that it's a form that's modified and weakened.

"It's like most treatments, in that the benefits outweigh – but don't diminish – the risks, Jean. But BCG has an excellent track record when it comes to preventing certain kinds of bladder cancer from coming back. Max is at high risk for a recurrence."

Dr. P glanced at the papers in Jean's hand and knew what was coming. He'd had plenty of patients do research on the Internet and in fact encouraged them to do so, as long as they were using reputable websites.

They talked some more, even weighing the idea of getting a second opinion, but in the end, Max and Jean decided to go ahead with the BCG treatments

The doctor gave the stack of papers back to Jean. "You'll have to tell your son-in-law about Quackwatch. He'll like that site."

"What is it? A list of phony doctors?" Max joked.

"Sort of. It's a website, www.quackwatch.org, that exposes health-related fraud, whether it's the sale of untested medicines or websites that don't have good information."

"I love it. For once, I'll have something to tell that son-in-law of mine about the Internet instead of him telling me," said Max.

Max's BCG treatments went well. He experienced some flulike symptoms after each treatment and felt a burning sensation in his bladder that became quite uncomfortable at times, but as Max said, "It was no sweat."

A Few Months Later

Max's first checkup was fine. But a few months later, he saw blood in his urine again. He stared for a moment. Then he went out to the porch and gazed out at the lilac bush that had just bloomed.

"I might not see that bush bloom again," Max thought. He knew that the blood might represent bad news. It could mean that his cancer had come back, and this time it might not have such a good outcome. On the other hand, he hoped, it might be just a urinary infection or some sort of late side effect of the immunotherapy.

Max waited until after Jean's birthday the next day to tell her that he'd had a problem. The doctor wanted to do a urinalysis and to see him right away. She, too, knew it might be serious.

When the urinalysis showed microscopic traces of blood in Max's urine, Dr. P scheduled him for an IVP, a bone scan, and an MRI.

> When the urinalysis showed microscopic traces of blood in Max's urine, Dr. P scheduled him for an IVP, a bone scan, and an MRI.

"You were right, Max," the doctor said when all the test results were in. "Your cancer has come back, but the good news is that it has not spread outside the bladder."

"What does that mean? Is it curable? Or should I take Jean on a cruise to Tahiti and spend all our retirement money?"

He laughed and said "No, Max. Better hang onto the retirement fund." A cure was still very possible in Max's case.

"Okay, Doc. What's next? Let's get going and see if we can kill this damn cancer once and for all."

Round Two

First came the chemo. This time it was different, given by injection rather than by catheter. Max went through three months of treatments that left him tired and 10 pounds lighter. On one occasion he even had a mouthful of sores that kept him from eating much solid food for a week after the treatments ended.

"Whoever thought I'd hate milkshakes?" Max reluctantly sipped a protein shake through a straw. "If I don't see another milkshake before I die, I won't be unhappy."

Then came the cystectomy, which Max dreaded. The doctor explained that the prostate, bladder, and lymph nodes would be removed. As a result, Max wouldn't be able to ejaculate or have an erection. Just as upsetting to Max as not being able to have intercourse was the prospect of having to empty urine from an internal "bladder" or –worst of all! – from an external bag. The mere idea sent him into a blue funk. The doctor's assurances that there were things that could be done about erectile dysfunction and bladder-collection systems didn't help. Max spent a lot of time staring at the lilac bush over the summer, feeling as if everything that made his life worthwhile was slipping away. These days, even his jokes fell flat.

"Well, Jean, you won't be needing those slinky nightgowns anymore, so I was thinking that maybe I'd start buying you power tools for your birthdays instead."

Jean didn't laugh. She said, "Max, I'll just be glad to have you here for my birthdays. I couldn't care less about the sex stuff. Your hugs are all I need."

That was another thing that upset Max. Since the cancer had come back, everyone treated him like a fragile vase that had a crack in it. They talked to him in voices filled with gentle sadness.

One day shortly before he went in for his cystectomy, he blew up at his daughter Nancy and said, "Hey! I'm not dead yet and I have no intention of dying at all, so quit tiptoeing around acting as if I'm laid out in my casket in the living room."

Max's outburst cleared the air and the tiptoeing eased up. The cloud of worry and fear lifted a little in Max's heart, too, and he realized that Jean was right: Being alive and able to embrace each other was what counted. He was wasting good time, moping around staring at a lilac bush. So he might not be able to take a leak anymore? Was that such a big deal? He never did like using public urinals and Jean wouldn't complain that he dripped on the floor or the toilet seat.

Reconstruction

Dr. P told Max that he was a good candidate for a neobladder, which meant that Dr. P's team would create an internal bladder that connected with Max's "internal plumbing," enabling him to void urine in a normal fashion.

"We may find during surgery that the neobladder isn't going to work for you, Max, in which case we'll do an internal pouch that you manually empty of urine."

The surgery took about four hours, and when Jean saw him in the recovery room, she told him he looked like a plate of spaghetti.

"You've got tubes everywhere! Down your nose, in your side, in your neck … a urine collection tube … and heaven knows what else."

Max groaned and drifted back to sleep. For the next four days, he was fed through the nasal tube while he healed. He didn't mind the tube, but he sure got hungry! To his surprise, he was up and walking … not far, but a few steps … the day after his surgery, tubes, bags, and all.

Each day Max got stronger and after a few days, the nurses told him to let them know the instant he felt the urge to urinate. Finally it came. He was taking his morning stroll down the hall and had to hurry back to his room, but he didn't mind. He knew it meant that he was healing and the neobladder was working.

One by one the tubes came out and the nurses taught Max how to catheterize himself so that he could flush out the bladder on a regular basis.

After 11 days in the hospital, all the tubes were out and Dr. P told Max that he could go home. He took a supply of protective underwear – which he called his training pants – home with him as well as a waterproof mattress pad in case the new bladder leaked.

"Sometimes you'll experience some leakage, Max – especially at night – until you learn to control the process. It's a little different from what you're used to. You have to train yourself to feel things differently and use your muscles differently. Just keep doing your exercises!"

The exercises were nothing more than a series of squeezes in the pelvic area, designed to make the muscles that controlled urination stronger. For some reason Max didn't like doing them. However, if it got him out of the training pants, he'd squeeze double-time.

It took Max a month or so before he felt "back to normal." His appetite was good, he didn't have to take an antibiotic anymore, and his bowels were functioning again. He still needed the protective underwear at night, but he found that he didn't mind it because he was wearing his regular boxers during the day.

Max's first-year checkup was clean. The CT scan showed no cancer. No metastasis. And Max hadn't had any symptoms.

After his second-year checkup, Max stood on the porch and looked at the lilac bush and smiled. The branches were loaded with blooms ready to burst into flower. Max knew the worry that his cancer might come back probably wouldn't ever leave him. But he finally felt that he could say with some confidence, "I am bladder-cancer survivor."

LIVING WITH CANCER

Cancer transforms everyone it touches; many cancer survivors describe their experience as a deep and motivating change. They find that what was "normal" during their pre-cancer lives no longer applies. Some say that life seems sweeter, that they are embracing life with a gusto and appreciation they didn't have before. Others feel the shadow of worry that their cancer might return, and some are gripped by guilt that they survived cancer while others were not so lucky.

Sometimes cancer survivors are quick to view their personal triumph over their disease as a benchmark for handling anything that might come their way in life, including a recurrence. Others who neither surge with confidence nor shake their fists at fate gradually return to a happier outlook, their faith in their health increasing along with hopes for the future.

Being diagnosed with cancer often gives people the feeling that they have no control. Survivorship is all about learning to take control over how you live the rest of your life.

What can you do to help keep yourself buoyed in your evolving role as a cancer survivor? Here are some tips from cancer survivors.

Start or return to an exercise routine. Research has shown that besides the physical benefits of exercise, the chemicals (endorphins) produced by your body during exercise can help you maintain a positive outlook.

Eat healthfully. Learning about food and nutrition is easy these days. From websites to magazines and cookbooks to television programs, a wealth of information and countless recipes are readily available. Ask your doctor for recommendations.

Stay connected to life. Survivors say that hobbies, friends, cherished pets, group activities, travel, and social activities all can help you get (or stay) involved in life.

Stay connected to your spirit. Whether you are religious or not, surviving cancer seems to awaken in many people an increased appreciation for the spiritual. Walking in the woods, listening to the ocean's waves, working in the garden, spending time with your grandchildren, or attending services at your church all can nurture your spirit.

Keep in touch with your medical team. While it's not healthy to worry about every ache or pain you experience, knowing when your body feels "different" is a clue that you need to talk to your doctor. In addition, it's important to follow a regular schedule of checkups – with your oncologist, primary care doctor, and even your dentist and eye doctor.

Take small steps. Sometimes the journey from cancer back to wholeness and health can be slow. Your body, your relationships, even your finances may have changed. Be patient with yourself and those around you. Let yourself gradually come to the belief that, like Max, you are indeed a survivor. ◆

WALKING THE LABYRINTH

Labyrinth walking is increasingly popular among those who seek a spiritual connection. It's offered in many senior centers, churches, hospitals, and centers such as The Gathering Place in Cleveland, a nonprofit community center for those touched by cancer (www.touchedbycancer.org).

Labyrinth walking can be as simple as following a route chalked out on the floor of a community room or as elaborate as a maze constructed of shrubs or stones or room dividers. Regardless of the layout of the labyrinth, your focus is on having a meaningful experience. Many people refer to the labyrinth as a "walking meditation."

Check with the resource center at your hospital, or ask your social worker or doctor about information on where to find opportunities in your area for labyrinth walking. While this is not a technique of *proven* benefit, it just might be helpful as an aid to calming you.

Chapter 5

Invasive Bladder Cancer

The word "invasive" refers to whether cells from your bladder cancer have "invaded" the muscle wall of the bladder, and if so, how far into the layers of muscle tissue it has penetrated. This can usually be determined from biopsy results, or occasionally when an operation has been performed to remove the bladder and some of the surrounding tissues. In some cases, organs near the bladder (such as the vagina in women, or the prostate in men) may have been invaded as well.

Invasive cancer extends further into the body than superficial TCC does and is therefore a more serious stage of the disease. It requires more complicated treatment, such as surgical removal of the bladder. This may, in turn, change how you manage basic physical functions in your everyday life, such as your bathroom habits and even your sex life. Also of importance is the significant rate of recurrence connected with invasive cancer. Often other organs, such as the lymph nodes, lung or liver, are involved.

Despite such a gloomy introduction to this chapter, there is every reason for you to be hopeful if you've been diagnosed with invasive cancer. Current treatment, which includes surgery (cystectomy), chemotherapy, radiation therapy, or two of these approaches combined, offers you an excellent chance for long-term survival and, in many cases, for a cure. This applies particularly to those invasive tumors that have not penetrated outside the bladder, the so-called "organ-confined" tumors.

There is no question that the after effects of surgical removal of the bladder (cystectomy) can be unsettling to think about. You won't have a bladder or maybe even a urethra any longer. How will you be able to pass urine? Will you have to have some type of urine-collecting bag? Will there be an odor? Will it show when you wear certain clothing?

We'll talk about all those things in more detail, but in brief, your team will need to surgically create an artificial urine-collection system for you. This is known as a urinary diversion system. In years past, the only option was a urine-collection bag worn outside the body, which many people found to be unpleasant or even embarrassing.

The good news is that now, in many cases, an artificial bladder (sometimes called a neobladder) can be fashioned from a piece taken from the intestine (bowel), enabling you to void urine in a normal or near-normal fashion. You'll have to learn to use a different set of muscles when urinating, and there may be some leakage now and then, particularly at night. Leakage can be controlled by wearing underwear designed with a disposable pad or, for men, a sort of condom. Overall, it's a more attractive option that makes it easier to face a complicated and often scary surgery such as cystectomy. And with modern techniques, most patients no longer have to contend with urinary leakage, except on rare occasions.

Even if you are disappointed because the creation of an internal urinary diversion system is not possible in your situation, keep in mind that there is also no question that cystectomy is a powerful weapon against invasive bladder cancer that can increase your odds of living a long, cancer-free life.

WHAT IS A CYSTECTOMY?

Cystectomy is the most common treatment option for invasive bladder cancer. In most cases, your medical team will recommend a complete (or radical) cystectomy. This means that your bladder, the lymph nodes tucked around your bladder in the abdomen, the prostate in men, and the uterus, ovaries, and part of the vaginal wall in women will be surgically removed. Depending on where the cancer is located, the urethra may also be removed.

It's easy to confuse some of the terms your doctors use, such as "cystoscopy" (a diagnostic procedure that introduces a tube into the bladder so that the doctor can look at the inner surface and take a biopsy) and "cystectomy" (the surgical removal of the bladder). Don't hesitate to ask your doctors for clarification.

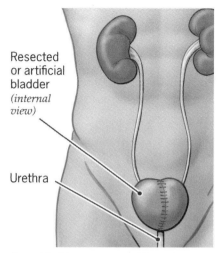

Resected or artificial bladder *(internal view)*

Urethra

A neobladder constructed from the intestine allows normal collection and voiding of urine without manual emptying of a pouch or reservoir.

Cystectomy seems like a drastic surgery, doesn't it? Why remove so many body parts? Why not just take the tumor and some surrounding tissue?

Depending on where your tumor is located, the cancer-causing substances responsible for the tumors in your bladder were also filtered through the kidney, ureters, and urethra, and there is a possibility that tumors may be forming in those organs, too. In particular, the tissues lining the bladder, ureters, and urethra (known as the urothelial tissues) may be at risk from the after effects of cancer-causing substances, such as agents in cigarette smoke or industrial dyes. Also, because your cancer may have penetrated the muscle wall, it's possible that organs surrounding the bladder, such as the prostate, uterus, or vagina, may also be at risk from further growth of the cancer cells.

So in the case of bladder cancer, which often recurs or spreads to other organs, you'll have a much better chance of a cure once organs and tissue have been removed in areas where the disease is likely to spread or where it may already have infiltrated. And a cure is what you and your doctors most definitely want to strive for.

Sometimes, if the cancer is very localized and surrounded by plenty of healthy, noncancerous tissue, a partial cystectomy might be recommended, whereby only a portion of the bladder is removed and some or all of the surrounding organs may be saved.

You probably have already figured out that cystectomy is a surgical procedure performed under anesthesia in a hospital setting. Depending on what kind of bladder reconstruction you have, you may stay in the hospital anywhere from 5 to 14 days.

The descriptions included here of medical procedures and treatments are of a general nature; your own experience may differ from what is discussed here.

With cystectomy, an incision is made through the abdominal wall, so you can expect some mild discomfort at the incision site. The incision will be covered, and you probably won't be able to shower or get the incision wet for about a week to 10 days. You may have a drain from the incision, a flexible tube with a hollow bulb on the end that you will remove, empty, flush out, and reattach as needed. Your doctor will remove the drain (it's painless) and any stitches or staples in a follow-up visit 10 days or so after your surgery.

Some possible complications include infection, bleeding, blood clots, or intestinal obstruction. You may experience some difficulties with your urinary diversion system. (See the section about urinary diversion systems later in this chapter.)

You'll be asked to wait for a few weeks after surgery before you drive, and your doctors are likely to want you to refrain for several weeks from doing anything that strains the abdominal area, such as pushing and pulling a vacuum cleaner or lifting heavy objects or engaging in any other activity that might damage the scar or even pull the scar tissue apart, thereby risking the formation of a hernia. A hernia occurs when your surgical scar pulls apart under the skin and allows a part of the underlying bowel to poke forward, creating a noticeable lump. It can interfere with the functioning of your bowel and therefore needs to be fixed, either with an external truss or support, or possibly through another surgical operation.

It's smarter just to avoid the risk in the first place by not stressing the scar soon after surgery. This is the time to take it easy and when possible allow friends or family to pamper you by helping with chores and housework. Just don't get too used to having someone bring you the morning newspaper and a cup of coffee! Generally it's a good idea to talk about this with your doctor and find out what you can and cannot safely do.

There are some negative consequences of cystectomy that you should discuss thoroughly with your medical team. As mentioned above, there may be changes in urinary function. These will depend largely on the type of surgery and on whether an artificial bladder has been created.

Sometimes while the abdominal tissues are healing after surgery there will be a period of irregular bowel function, during which you will unexpectedly have to deal with diarrhea or constipation.

Occasionally there will be some swelling in one or both legs, due either to fluid retention or the formation of scar tissue around the lymph vessels that drain the legs.

Often there will be the presence of an asymptomatic, low-grade chronic urinary tract infection that will be identified upon routine testing. This occurs because of the changed pattern of emptying the new bladder. Usually it causes no problems and doesn't require active treatment with antibiotics.

Other issues also arise. Worries about possible changes in sexual function are common, and very normal. Sexual function often does change after cystectomy. That doesn't mean you can't have an active, playful, pleasurable sex life with your partner. It does mean that you'll probably explore innovative strategies as you seek comfortable ways to experience fulfillment.

Men experience more extreme changes in sexual function after surgery than women do. Around half the men who undergo cystectomy experience nerve damage that leaves them impotent afterwards, a serious lifestyle change that is not only physical but emotional, requiring much thoughtful discussion between you, your partner, and your medical team both before surgery and after.

If you are able to have an erection after surgery, you won't be able to ejaculate, because without a prostate, your body is no longer able to produce semen. You'll find that the physical sensation of orgasm is different from what you are accustomed to. It's not unpleasant; just different. In general, the younger you are at the time of surgery, the more likely you will be to have erections or to regain over time the capability of having them. There are surgical procedures, such as penile inserts, that can help make sexual activity possible.

For women, a cystectomy includes the removal of the uterus and part of the vaginal wall. What does that mean for you?

Well, for one thing, your vagina may be narrower as a result of the surgery. Usually it's possible to continue to have intercourse, although sometimes there can be some pain involved. Be sure to talk to your doctor if you do experience pain as there are methods of reducing this.

Most women diagnosed with bladder cancer already have experienced menopause. (Typically, women who receive diagnoses of bladder cancer are older.) For younger women, that may not be the case. The removal of the uterus and possibly of other female organs near the bladder brings an abrupt end to the childbearing years. It may also set off typical menopausal symptoms such as hot flashes or mood swings if the ovaries have been removed at surgery (removal of ovaries is unusual). If you find yourself feeling depressed or blue or uncomfortable from hot flashes, talk to your doctor. You don't have to feel that way; there are options available for you to consider.

> Most women diagnosed with bladder cancer already have experienced menopause. (Typically, women who receive diagnoses of bladder cancer are older.)

As is recommended for men, talking with your partner and your medical team about the physical and emotional changes that you may experience after a cystectomy is an important part of the process, one that deserves as much consideration as the more immediate decisions about which treatment options you want to pursue.

Keep in mind that cystectomy is a life-preserving weapon against invasive cancer. That doesn't mean you can't or shouldn't consider the possibility of impotence or altered sexual function with your partner, or the inability to carry a child. It does offer the hope that you can celebrate many more years of healthy, loving life with your friends and family. That's an important thing to remember at a time when life may seem to be serving you big helpings of despair.

STRATEGIES FOR DAILY
LIFE AFTER CYSTECTOMY

- Drink lots of water. If you have a neobladder or reservoir formed from your intestine, mucus will continue to be excreted from the intestinal tissue and must be "flushed" regularly to prevent infection. Regular consumption of fluids helps flush out the mucus.

- Maintain good personal hygiene in bathroom habits, hand-washing, and/or the care and cleaning of your stoma or reservoir.

- If you have an external pouch, change it daily.

- Learn to recognize the signs of infection, including vomiting, nausea, poor appetite, fever, pain in the back, and strong-smelling or stinking urine.

- Exercise. Did you do aerobics before your cystectomy? Play tennis? Run marathons? You still can. And you should.

- If you're feeling blue, talk to someone. Your doctor, nurse, social worker, spouse, a good friend, and your pastor are all good candidates.

- Take some time for yourself. Listen to music, read a book, take a walk, bake cookies, wash the car, get a manicure ... Whatever relaxes you, make time to do it.

- If your sexual function has changed, don't be afraid to explore different patterns of intimacy. There are many ways to satisfy a partner, many ways to achieve a close and loving relationship. If you and your partner are uncomfortable discussing this side of your relationship, perhaps talking to your doctor or nurse or social worker individually is an option. Whatever your age, you're too young to give up a loving relationship.

- Don't strive for perfection. Just for now, until you've regained your physical strength and the emotional roller coaster has slowed, go easy on the expectations you set for yourself. Let others help, or let the chores go for a while.

CONTINENT URINARY DIVERSION SYSTEMS

Sometimes an internal bladder connected to the urethra (the tube that carries urine to the outside of the body) isn't possible and you will instead have a continent urinary diversion system. This means that you'll have a pouch or reservoir, either external or more commonly internal, that collects your urine, and you'll have to empty the pouch. This is also known as an ostomy or ileal conduit system.

Pouch (internal)

Stoma (external)

With a continent urinary diversion system, the urine is collected and stored in a pouch inside the body, and emptied manually through the stoma several times a day.

The more common continent urinary diversion system is an **internal reservoir**, or pouch, made from a piece of intestine. The pouch is inside your body, but you must manually empty and flush the reservoir by inserting a syringe or catheter into a permanent "hole" or stoma in your abdomen. Often the stoma is located unobtrusively in your navel, where it is not likely to be detected by a casual glance.

Your doctor, may, however, recommend an **external pouch** that is situated outside your body and attaches to your abdomen through a "hole" or stoma. You must manually empty the external pouch and cleanse the stoma.

Either alternative sounds unpleasant, but having a pouch (particularly an internal reservoir) won't interfere with your life or self-image as much as you might expect, if at all.

You can still snorkel and swim. You can dance in a clingy, swingy dress or bike in Spandex shorts. You can do your job, whether it's manning a drill press or managing a Fortune 500 company. And you can still look and feel sexy and enjoy a satisfying intimate relationship with your partner.

How is that possible with a pouch of urine attached to your body? Won't it leak or smell?

No, it shouldn't. It won't take you long to adapt to emptying the pouch. Keeping it clean and emptied is the key to feeling – and being – fresh. You'll discover that you can enjoy a glass of wine at a party and excuse yourself a short time later to empty the pouch and freshen up without anyone knowing you have an ostomy system.

External pouches are designed to lie flat against your body and

Stoma (external)

Reservoir (internal)

With an ileal conduit system, an external pouch is worn to collect urine and is emptied manually. The pouch connects to the body at the stoma, which empties urine into the pouch as it is collected in the reservoir.

can be discreetly worn under most clothing (even "body shaping" underwear for women or athletic supporters for men). There are different sizes of pouches as well, along with waterproof or protective coverings. Internal reservoirs are even easier to conceal.

You're probably still not convinced that you can look and feel as feminine or masculine as you did without a pouch or reservoir.

For example, what do you do when your partner wants to have sex? What if your pouch leaks or becomes dislodged during an intimate moment?

There are lines of intimate apparel, some quite sensual, others very practical, that are designed with special protective concealed pockets for your pouch. You can look and feel downright sexy without worrying. Really.

The Wound Ostomy and Continence Nurses Society maintains a website at www.wocn.org (1-888-224-9626). The site offers lots of information and a list of apparel companies. One such line of apparel is Intimate Moments, found on the web at www.intimatemoments apparel.com (1-201-825-9931).

Your nurse and doctor can give you lots of tips and instructions. Don't hesitate to talk to them and ask questions. You'll want to know what the signs of infection are, whether there are any restrictions on your activities (for example, some contact sports are restricted), and what diet or exercise constraints you might have.

Give yourself time to adjust. Life can be – and usually is – just fine, in spite of having a pouch.

> **DID YOU KNOW THAT?**
>
> Certain foods, such as asparagus and some seafood, give your urine a strong odor. You might want to avoid those foods if you're going to be at a party or out in public.

TREATMENT RAMIFICATIONS

One of the difficult issues for you and your medical team is to work out exactly what to do about the treatment of invasive bladder cancer. It is clear that cystectomy can be a life-saving procedure, yet many patients with invasive bladder cancer still eventually die of the disease, especially if it has penetrated the surrounding organs.

Your team will make a recommendation about treatment after carefully evaluating such very important factors as the extent of invasion by tumor cells (the stage), the normal or disorganized/abnormal appearance of the cancer cells under the microscope (grade), whether the cancer cells have invaded lymphatic channels or blood vessels, whether cancer cells are growing within the lymph nodes, and whether a specific cell control gene called P53 is normal.

If your cancer is organ-confined (i.e., if the cancer cells have not spread beyond the boundaries of the bladder and its immediate surrounding tissues), if it has not penetrated beyond the first layers of surrounding muscle, if there is no lymphatic or vascular invasion, and if lymph nodes are negative (i.e., they contain no cancer cells), the chance of permanent cure by cystectomy alone is around 80 percent.

If, however, your cancer has penetrated deeply into the muscle or has a very poor level of cellular organization (high grade), if the P53 gene has mutated, or if invasion of lymphatic tissues or blood vessels ("lympho-vascular invasion") is present, the chance of permanent cure may be much lower. In general, if things go badly after cystectomy, the problem is that cancer cells show themselves in other parts of the body (metastases) – a very dangerous situation.

Over the past half-century, doctors have tried many approaches to improving the results, including the use of radiotherapy or the combination of radiotherapy and cystectomy. Neither of these approaches appears to have provided the solution.

Since the 1950s it has been known that cancer-killing drugs (chemotherapy) can sometimes shrink bladder cancer that has spread through the body, and sometimes they can completely eliminate the deposits of cancer in different parts of the body. In the past 25 years, several studies have looked at the impact of combining chemotherapy with cystectomy or with radiotherapy in an attempt to improve survival figures. Before that discussion, let's talk a bit about chemotherapy.

CHEMOTHERAPY

Chemotherapy is a term that refers to the use of drugs to kill cancer cells. Chemotherapy is usually given by intravenous injection (injection by needle directly into the vein), but sometimes it can be administered as a tablet or even through a urinary catheter (intravesical) for a patient with superficial bladder cancer. (See Chapter 4.) There are many different types of chemotherapy, and a detailed discussion is beyond the scope of this book. Your medical team will talk with you about what type of chemotherapy is best for you and why.

In brief, chemotherapy drugs mostly act to interfere with the ability of cancer cells to divide and multiply, often by inhibiting the function of enzymes within the cells or by blocking cell division and the formation of RNA and DNA, the substances of life. Because these drugs act on cells that are dividing and multiplying, they can also affect some normal tissues and thus can cause a range of side effects. Common side effects you might experience may include nausea and/or vomiting, hair loss, suppression of the bone marrow (bone marrow forms the blood; its suppression may cause increased risk of fatigue, infection or bleeding), and occasionally specific reactions to individual drugs (such as allergic reactions and lung inflammation).

Keep your doctor informed if you are experiencing any of the above side effects. There are drugs that can help minimize these conditions and make your treatment more comfortable. Luckily, these side effects tend to disappear once you are no longer receiving chemotherapy, and you will gradually feel stronger and become less vulnerable to bleeding or infections.

For invasive bladder cancer, chemotherapy is sometimes given before you have a cystectomy. Sometimes it's given afterwards. Sometimes it's not given at all. It depends entirely on the type of tumor you have, where it may have spread, and whether you have another medical condition that might make it difficult for you to tolerate chemotherapy. Very advanced age can also be a factor in deciding whether chemotherapy is appropriate.

The choice of drugs used to treat invasive bladder cancer is similar to the choice in advanced or metastatic disease, and we will cover that in Chapter 6. If you have invasive transitional cell carcinoma you will probably undergo chemotherapy, as this type of cancer is responsive to either radiotherapy or surgery with chemotherapy, and many studies have examined this type of cancer treatment.

If you have been diagnosed with squamous cell cancer or adenocarcinoma, the track record for chemotherapy is not so clearly defined. Most physicians don't recommend chemotherapy as *standard* treatment in conjunction with cystectomy for these types of cancer. It is, however, quite reasonable for your team to suggest that you look into a clinical trial (for example, one that is exploring the use of chemotherapy) if you have been diagnosed with squamous cell or adenocarcinoma. (Clinical trials are not "standard" care and will be discussed in Chapter 6.)

For invasive transitional cell carcinoma, most of the information from clinical trials has been obtained from patients who were initially given chemotherapy by intravenous injection and who then went on to cystectomy or to definitive radiotherapy. (More on that later.)

Most of the reported trials indicate that the use of single chemotherapy drugs does not have an extensive beneficial effect, but that the use of combinations of three or four chemotherapy drugs can shrink the bladder cancer in around 70 percent of cases and can also improve the cure rate and length of survival.

For you as a patient, the information gleaned from these clinical trials means that if you have TCC, your doctors are likely to recommend treatment that includes a "cocktail" of several carefully targeted chemotherapy drugs as well as cystectomy or radiotherapy.

In some cancers, such as breast cancer, it is pretty standard practice to give several doses of chemotherapy *after* surgery, especially for tumors with high-risk pathological features, such as lymph-node involvement. We know of six studies that have looked at this question in bladder cancer, but the results are somewhat inconclusive as to whether chemotherapy is most effective given before or after surgery.

CARES AT CLEVELAND CLINIC

Scott Hamilton, an Olympic gold medalist in figure skating, is a survivor of testicular cancer. The experience of being diagnosed and treated successfully for cancer at Cleveland Clinic in 1997 led Scott to dedicate his life to promoting cancer research and awareness.

With Cleveland Clinic Taussig Cancer Institute, he established the Scott Hamilton CARES Initiative (Cancer Alliance for Research, Education and Survivorship) for patients and their families. One of CARES' ongoing projects is the 4th Angel mentoring program, which pairs newly diagnosed cancer patients with people who have been through similar experiences of cancer and cancer treatment. (See Chapter 7 for more on the 4th Angel program.)

CARES also is the home of www.chemocare.com, Scott's website for people anticipating chemotherapy treatment. It's jam-packed with tips on dealing with chemo, how to manage side effects, drug information, and much more.

There is a large randomized trial in progress in Europe that will tell doctors whether intravenous chemotherapy after cystectomy improves the cure rate. Until the results of that study are available, most medical teams recommend consideration of first-line chemotherapy, followed by cystectomy for deeply invasive bladder cancer. Sometimes a cystectomy reveals a cancer that is deeper or more extensive than had been expected; in that situation, the urologist or oncologist will usually discuss the benefits and drawbacks of using chemotherapy (so-called "adjuvant chemotherapy"), typically with the same drugs that might have been given before surgery. (See Chapter 6.)

SOME CHEMOTHERAPY COMBINATIONS AND SIDE EFFECTS

Below are some common chemotherapy combinations. This is not an exhaustive list by any means. Talk with your doctor about your treatment plan. Remember that not all people experience all side effects. Your general health, age, other drugs you might be taking, and the dosage of the chemotherapy drugs may affect what side effects you experience. Many side effects are unpleasant but are temporary, and the severity of these effects is highly variable. Some side effects are more serious and you should talk with your medical team about them.

*In the bulleted items on pages 91 and 92, * represents more serious side effects.*

MVAC: METHOTREXATE, VINBLASTINE, DOXORUBICIN (ADRIAMYCIN), CISPLATIN

This is usually given in four to six cycles of 28 days. The typical treatment is to administer methotrexate on day 1 and vinblastine, doxorubicin, and cisplatin on day 2. Then boosters of methotrexate and vinblastine are given on days 15 and 22, and the cycle begins again on day 29. Administration of methotrexate is separated from that of cisplatin by a day as the two drugs have the potential to interact adversely, causing damage to the kidneys; also, cisplatin sometimes slows excretion of methotrexate through the kidneys. Regular blood tests are made during treatment. If MVAC is used as adjuvant or neo-adjuvant therapy, only three cycles are given in most programs of treatment.

Common side effects, which most people experience, include:

- Fatigue
- Interference with bone-marrow function, which can cause risk of infections, tiredness, shortness of breath, bruises, nosebleeds or bleeding gums, and mouth sores*
- Changes in liver or kidney function (determined by blood tests)*
- Inability to hear high-pitched sounds, ringing in the ears, and/or blurred vision
- Nausea and/or vomiting*
- Possible harm to unborn child and/or infertility (uncommon in this patient population because of age)*
- Temporary hair loss (usually a complete loss of body hair, which may start about three to six weeks after treatment begins)
- Sensitivity to sunlight
- Pink or red urine for a day or two after treatment

Less common side effects include:

- Temporary irregular heartbeat*
- Redness, stinging, burning, or leakage around the needle/drip site
- Skin rash or itching, dizziness, or headache during treatment (indicates allergic reaction – tell your nurse immediately)*
- Loss of appetite, metallic taste in mouth
- Diarrhea or constipation (if either continues more than three days, talk with your doctor)
- Tingling or numbness in hands or feet
- Coughing or shortness of breath
- Eyes watery or irritated for a few days after treatment

CMV: CISPLATIN, METHOTREXATE, VINBLASTINE

This is usually given in four cycles of three-week courses. Regular blood tests are made during treatment. On day 1, vinblastine and methotrexate are administered, usually on an outpatient basis. On day 2, cisplatin is administered, sometimes with an overnight stay (especially in the case of an older patient or one who is less healthy).

Common side effects, which many people experience, include:

- Fatigue
- Interference with bone-marrow function, which can cause risk of infection, tiredness, shortness of breath, bruises, nosebleeds, or bleeding gums*
- Temporary hair loss or thinning (this may start about three to four weeks after your treatment begins)
- Kidney damage (determined by blood tests)*
- Inability to hear high-pitched sounds, ringing in the ears, and/or blurred vision
- Nausea and/or vomiting*
- Possible harm to unborn child and/or infertility (unlikely in most bladder-cancer patients because of their age)*

Less common (occasional) side effects include:

- Redness, stinging, burning, or leakage around the needle/drip site
- Skin rash or itching, dizziness, headache during treatment (indicates allergic reaction – tell your nurse immediately)*
- Loss of appetite, metallic taste in mouth
- Diarrhea or constipation (if either continues more than three days, talk with your doctor)
- Sensitivity to sunlight
- Tingling or numbness in hands or feet
- Coughing or shortness of breath

WHAT IS CHEMO FOG?

If you've been undergoing chemotherapy, you may have noticed that you're having trouble remembering things – even simple things like your phone number – and you may not be able to concentrate enough to finish your usual morning crossword.

It might be a side effect of your chemo, one that has been dubbed "chemo fog" or "chemo brain."

Most of the time the "brain fuzziness" that can be a side effect of chemotherapy is short-lived and improves rapidly after treatment ends, usually within six months. But sometimes it doesn't.

Some patients have reported that their cognitive (thought) impairment lasts for months or even years after chemotherapy has ended. And sometimes the fuzziness is more than just forgetting a phone number. It can be an inability to understand basic math or a crippling inability to remember how to perform certain tasks, and it can cause great difficulty as you endeavor to carry out duties at work and at home. Fortunately this type of severe problem is extremely uncommon.

Chemo fog seems to be more common in patients who have received large doses of chemo drugs, but researchers aren't sure why some people are affected or how much chemotherapy it takes to cause impairment. Chemo fog is being studied by a number of researchers and is becoming a recognized problem among physicians and patients.

Talk to your doctor about any problems that you experience with memory or concentration. There are memory-training exercises and strategies that can help your memory or reasoning skills. Some recent research suggests that prescribed stimulants may lessen the effects.

Talk openly with your family, friends, and loved ones about problems you experience with chemo fog. Once they are aware of the problem, you may feel less isolated and inept. And it can open the door for everyone to approach the problem with compassion and a sense of humor.

GEM-CIS: GEMCITABINE, CISPLATIN

This treatment is usually administered on an outpatient basis. A blood test and saline drip are required before each treatment. The course of treatment usually proceeds in four to six cycles of 21 days (or alternatively on a 28-day cycle), with cisplatin and gemcitabine administered on day 1, gemcitabine only on day 8, with the cycle repeating on day 21. Sometimes an extra dose of gemcitabine is given on day 15, in which case the cycle repeats at day 28.

Common side effects include:

- Risk of infection (contact your physician immediately if you suddenly feel very ill or your temperature goes above 100 degrees)
- Bruising, bleeding, anemia, tiredness
- Nausea*
- Rash, itchiness, swelling in the ankles
- Loss of appetite or food tastes unpleasant; diarrhea
- Tingling or numbness in hands and/or feet*
- Drowsiness*

Less common side effects include:

- Ringing in the ears or other hearing difficulties
- Thinning hair (hair loss is less likely with GEM-CIS)
- Coughing, shortness of breath*
- Possible harm to unborn child and/or infertility (uncommon in this patient population because of age)*

RADIOTHERAPY (RADIATION)

Radiation uses radioactive beams or pellets to kill cancer cells. Your medical team may recommend a course of radiation therapy in addition to chemotherapy and/or surgery.

The most common way to give radiation therapy for bladder cancer uses an invisible external beam delivered through a machine that focuses it on the area that requires treatment. You'll find that it's painless and that the experience is similar to having an ordinary x-ray done. In the usual approach, your doctors will use your CT scan as a roadmap of the abdomen and pelvis to set up a "line" for the beam that pinpoints your tumor. In another type of radiotherapy, doctors implant a small pellet or needle of radioactive material directly into your cancer. (This is rarely used for bladder cancer these days.)

When radiation is used alone or with chemotherapy, there is an increased likelihood that your other organs, such as the prostate and uterus, will remain functional, as does your ability to void urine normally and have sex. The intention when chemotherapy and radio-therapy are given is usually to improve the chances of curing the cancer while preserving the bladder and avoiding the need to remove it surgically. This area is still somewhat controversial; while some physicians believe that this approach is nearly as effective as surgical removal of the bladder, others feel that cystectomy is the best treat-ment. The decision depends in part upon the physical fitness of the patient as well as upon the patient's personal preferences.

The use of radiotherapy doesn't mean that it is without side effects. There can be scarring of the bladder tissue, and that can reduce the amount of urine your bladder can hold. The result would be an increase in the number of times you have to urinate, which can be irritating, especially at night. You also may experience an increase in bouts of cystitis.

There has been much discussion about whether the results achieved by radiotherapy are the same as those from cystectomy with respect to achieving cure. We think that when one considers all types of bladder cancer, in the hands of a highly experienced urologist who specializes in this operation, cystectomy gives better results than radiotherapy. However, there are some patients, particularly those with other significant medical conditions, who will benefit from radiotherapy despite the possibility of a lower chance of permanent cure. In some centers, such as Massachusetts General Hospital, where the techniques of chemoradiotherapy and bladder preservation have been piloted, a urologist will perform a cystoscopy about halfway through the planned course of radiotherapy. If the tumor is shrinking well, radiotherapy will be completed. However, if it appears that the cancer is not responding to radiotherapy, the plan will be abandoned and replaced with a radical cystectomy.

WHAT HAPPENS NEXT?

There are no absolute guidelines for follow-up after cystectomy. What is right for you will depend on your situation: the type of urinary diversion system you have, whether you received chemotherapy and/or radiotherapy, and what, if any, side effects you are dealing with.

A reasonable guide for follow-up, however, is to have a physical exam, chest x-ray, urine test, and blood work every three months for the first year, every four months for the next two years, and then twice a year for life. We usually recommend an annual CT or MRI for the first five years at least.

As with superficial cancer, if you have any symptoms discussed in Chapter 1, check in with your doctor. Call him if you have blood in your urine or an increase in the urge or frequency of urination. It might just be an infection, but the best thing to do is to make contact without unnecessary delay.

Because you have had an invasive form of cancer, the chance that it may spread to other organs is more likely than with superficial cancer. And the sooner a recurrence or spread (metastasis) is discovered, the better chance you have of a satisfactory outcome. Therefore it's especially important to be aware of any changes in your body and to talk to your doctor about them right away.

Are you more tired than usual – not just today, but on a regular basis? Are you losing weight, even though you're eating more than your share of that chocolate ice cream in the freezer? Do you have any new aches in your muscles or bones, or perhaps a persistent headache?

Even if you have a checkup coming up in a few weeks, if you experience any of these signs or symptoms or even just have a vague feeling that something isn't right, don't wait. Call and talk to your doctor.

PREVENTION

Other than the strategies suggested in Chapter 4, there are no specific things you can do to avoid a recurrence or metastasis.

Being positive, living your life to the fullest without concern about whether your cancer will come back and whether you'll survive if it does recur, is an important approach to dealing with cancer and its after effects. However, it's sometimes harder to achieve than just willing yourself not to worry.

To brighten your outlook, activities, interests, and involvements are key. Play with your children, spend time with your spouse and friends, work at a job or hobby you love, nourish yourself through faith or spiritual contemplation, eat well, move and stretch your body as much as you are able, and take time to do at least some of the special things you've always thought about doing, whether it's as simple as taking a nap on your porch in the sunshine or learning to knit, or as complex as learning to sail. Above all else, DON'T SMOKE!

TREATMENT CASE STUDY: DIANE

It was Tuesday. Day No. 2 of Diane's MVAC chemotherapy cycle. She dreaded going, not because the process hurt or even because she felt fatigued and a little nauseated for a few days after her treatment, but because it took four or five hours to complete and today was a sunny, warm spring day. How much nicer to be outside doing just about anything, even pulling weeds in the garden, rather than sitting in the clinic, hooked up to a container of intravenous fluid running into her arm.

When she got to the clinic, she stopped at the lab to get a blood test. Before she could have her chemotherapy treatment, her doctors wanted to make sure that her blood results were within normal ranges. If anything – her kidney-function test, for example – were too abnormal, the treatment might have to be delayed while additional fluids were pushed through to flush her kidneys.

After her blood test, she headed for the chemo lounge and waited while the pharmacist assembled her treatment. The clinic was crowded and it took about half an hour before Diane's name was called.

"Isn't it depressing to go to chemo?" Diane's sister had asked when she came over that morning to drive Diane to her appointment.

"No. At least not usually. I like to think of it as a place of hope. Without those drugs, I'd have no way to fight this cancer. And I want to fight it."

It was Diane's lucky day. There were a number of recliner-style chairs in the chemo room, and Diane liked the ones upholstered in fabric rather than fake leather. They were softer and not so slippery. Today the blue chair was available – her favorite.

Paulette, one of the chemo nurses, threaded a fine tube called a cannula into a vein in Diane's forearm. It always hurt a little to have the line put in, sort of like a pinprick, but Paulette started talking about her son, who was trying to decide what college to go to, and before Diane knew it, the line was in.

The doctor had offered her the option of a central line, a permanent gadget also called a port, inserted under local anesthetic, that would sit just below the collarbone throughout the entire period of chemotherapy treatment. This would spare her the weekly intravenous sticks but it would make showering a bit more complicated, and she decided to try to avoid this choice in order to keep things as simple as possible. "I have pretty good veins," she thought, "and hopefully they will be okay for the duration of chemotherapy."

Paulette gave her a dose of anti-nausea drugs through the cannula and then started an infusion (also known as "a drip") of sterile salt water.

"I wish this part would go faster," said Diane.

"Thirty minutes isn't that long, and it's worth it. The kidneys need to soak up a good drink of salt water to keep the cisplatin from doing any damage. Cisplatin is dangerous for the kidneys, so we always flush it through them as quickly as is safe." Paulette patted Diane's hand. "Besides, I taped three episodes of *Monk* for you to watch today. How's that?"

Diane loved Adrian Monk, the obsessive-compulsive detective, and didn't get the program on any of her cable channels at home. Paulette did. "Hey, thanks."

By the time one episode of *Monk* was over, Paulette had already given the premedications (anti-nausea drugs and a type of cortisone to help Diane to tolerate the chemotherapy better) and had started administering the vinblastine and doxorubicin. They were colorless, and like the sterile salt water, took a little over half an hour to drip into Diane's system. Paulette was particularly careful when administering the doxorubicin; she had explained that it can be quite damaging to the skin and local tissues if it leaks out of the cannula or if the cannula is not placed properly in the vein.

Then came the cisplatin, also colorless, but this took almost two hours to slowly make its way into Diane's body. Diane always kidded that she'd have bedsores before the cisplatin was done dripping. When the *Monk* episodes were over, Diane tried to read, but as usual, she couldn't, so she closed her eyes and put on her headphones to listen to music.

Finally, after another hour of sterile salt-water (saline) drip, Diane's treatment was over. Paulette slid the cannula out and gave Diane a supply of anti-nausea drugs.

"You take these – every one, Diane – whether you think you need them or not. You hear me?" Paulette shook her finger. "It's easier to prevent feeling sick than it is to stop it once it gets hold of you." Diane regretted telling Paulette that after the previous treatment she hadn't taken the anti-nausea drugs because she felt fine.

Carl was waiting for her in the lounge.

"Another one down, baby," she said as she kissed him. "I can feel that wicked cisplatin chewing up those nasty little cancer cells."

Diane knew that she would probably crash once she got home. She hadn't slept well since she had started chemo because her feet tingled a lot, especially at night. It felt as if her feet had been asleep and were waking up.

Paulette told her that after her treatment ended the tingling would go away gradually over a period of weeks, along with the funny, almost metallic, taste in her mouth that Diane had all the time. The mouth rinse that the doctor had prescribed helped with the sores in her mouth, but not the funny taste.

"You're about average," Paulette had told her when Diane asked whether she was having more or fewer side effects than other patients experienced. "Maybe fewer – at least so far. Your hair's getting brittle. That's normal, too. Some things may get a little worse as we go along, though."

Diane didn't care what side effects she had or how tough it got. The feeling that the drugs were beating back the cancer gave her the strength to keep going.

She'd be back again, on days 15 and 22 of her treatment cycle, for a boost of methotrexate and vinblastine. Then there'd be a rest before the whole process started over again on day 29.

"One and a half cycles down, one and a half to go," Diane said to Carl. "I'll be glad when it's over."

Surgery

Four weeks after her chemo treatments finished, Diane went in for her cystectomy surgery.

Thank heavens the doctor had spent a lot of time preparing Diane for what it would be like after surgery. Otherwise, Diane thought, she would have been frightened to see tubes and drains and catheters coming out of her body when she woke up. And upset that she wouldn't be able to drink for a day or two or eat solid food for several days, until her bowel and urinary tract system were back to normal.

Some of the tubes and drains and catheters were connected to the site of the operation and to the internal urine pouch Dr. S had made from Diane's small intestine. The pouch was connected internally to the ureters, which drained urine from the kidneys into the pouch just as they would into a normal bladder. The difference was that once the pouch healed, it would have to be emptied manually. For the first few weeks, however, the pouch drained into a temporary external collecting bag through a catheter.

Diane couldn't wait to get rid of the external pouch but she was looking forward to going home even more. She begged the doctors to send her home a day earlier than planned.

"I just want all these tubes and drains out of my body. My hair is growing back and I want to go home and take a shower, and wear my own clothes and feel neat and clean and … normal."

Deep down, Diane knew that "normal" wouldn't be the same as before she was diagnosed with cancer, but she was determined that no one, not even Carl, would notice that there was anything different about how her body functioned. Emptying and flushing the pouch struck Diane as a messy and distasteful prospect and she didn't want to think about it, much less talk about it.

To her surprise, she found that once she got the hang of things, taking care of the pouch wasn't as unpleasant as she expected.

She drained the pouch five or six times a day and once or twice during the night by inserting a catheter into the stoma, or opening, in her navel and letting the urine drain from the internal pouch into the toilet. It took her a month or two to be able to recognize the feeling when the pouch was full of urine and needed to be emptied. It took even longer to learn to thread the catheter into the pouch smoothly and to feel when it was positioned properly in the pouch. The nurse who showed her how to use the catheter told her that sometimes rolling the tube between her fingers made it easier to insert, a trick that worked well for Diane. The nurse's advice to relax during the process wasn't quite so easy to follow.

After a few weeks of practice, Diane was able to manage the process rather well. She knew not to use Vaseline to lubricate the catheter. (But K-Y jelly was on the approved list and worked very well.) She could tell when she'd drained all the urine from the pouch, and she knew how to flush it with saline water once or twice a day. She drank lots of water during the day but not in the evening before bedtime. This helped control the stoma's mucus production, a natural function since the pouch and stoma were made from intestinal tissue.

She even learned a few tricks from talking to other patients in the waiting room. One woman told her how to protect her clothes from mucus by cutting ultra-thin maxi pads in half and taping them over the stoma. The same woman also suggested folding the catheter over on itself and pinching it shut before removing it from the pouch. That way urine wouldn't drain out onto her clothing.

"All in all, I'm managing," Diane told Carl two months after the surgery when he asked her how she was doing. "Better than I expected. I still feel like a freak sometimes, but I guess that goes with the territory. I'm not sure I'll ever feel comfortable with the pouch, but at least I'm getting over being worried that people might somehow be able to tell that I'm not normal."

"You're normal. Maybe not quite the same normal as the day you were born, but you're still normal, Diane. It's not like you have horns and three heads."

"No, just a maxi pad taped on my stomach."

"So what? My sister wears Depends. It's no different."

Diane laughed and gave him a kiss. "I guess it isn't. Thanks. That really makes me feel better."

Despite Carl's assurances, Diane worried that there might be an odor from the stoma, and she struggled with worry that her cancer would recur. After her first checkup went well, the worry eased a bit. It eased even more when her second, third, and fourth checkups all were clear.

"Life is good, huh?" said Carl. "We got over the problems early on when it hurt you to make love, and now it's been almost two years and you're still cancer-free."

Diane nodded. "You know, Carl, I don't worry about it coming back anymore, except right before I have to go in for my checkup. Then I get a queasy feeling and I always worry like crazy until Dr. H calls and says it's all good news. Then I go back to not thinking about it. Someone called me a survivor the other day, and it surprised me. I don't think of myself as a survivor, exactly. I think of myself as … lucky. Blessed with good health and determined to do everything I can to keep myself that way." ◆

Chapter 6

Advanced
Bladder Cancer

Despite prompt and appropriate medical treatment, if you have muscle-invasive TCC, there is about a 50 percent chance that your cancer will metastasize (spread), either to another organ in the body or within the bladder area itself.

The most common sites of "distant metastasis" (not in the immediate area of the bladder) are the para-aortic lymph nodes and the liver, lungs, and bone. Occasionally, bladder cancer can send deposits through the bloodstream to the brain, but usually this happens only after prolonged and repeated treatment. Most recurrences, both distant and local, occur within the first two years after treatment.

One point worth emphasizing is that cancer cells in a distant metastasis still have the characteristics of the bladder cancer (i.e., they behave in the pattern of those bladder-cancer cells and don't really constitute "bone cancer" or "liver cancer" as such). Thus the drugs that may work against bladder-cancer cells also have a chance of working against these metastases located at other sites in the body.

As you might expect, the metastasis of your cancer is a dangerous situation that reduces your chance of a permanent cure. That doesn't mean that cure is impossible or that you no longer have options. Some established chemotherapy approaches can sometimes achieve cure if the metastases are not too extensive. In addition, new and promising therapies, including novel chemotherapy drugs, are undergoing clinical trials as this book goes to print, and many of those may well be available to you.

Imaging can reveal whether the cancer has spread.

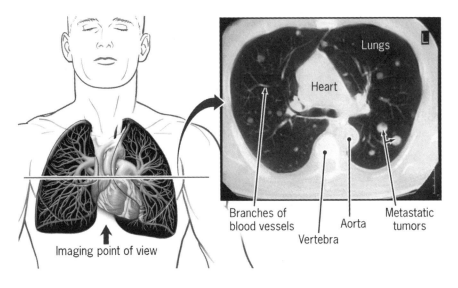

When metastasis occurs, the direction of your treatment shifts somewhat from a totally focused attempt to achieve cure. In this situation, while we attempt to cure the metastatic cancer if possible, we also try to palliate (reduce) the symptoms and we place a greater emphasis on comfort and pain control. This type of treatment is called palliative care. At this point, not only you but your family and loved ones should be involved with your medical team in understanding the progression of your disease and making decisions about your care.

This is a very important point and it can be confusing. On the one hand, your medical team is still trying very actively to cure the cancer, if possible, and to prolong your life and improve its quality to the maximum extent. However, as the chance of cure is somewhat smaller, you and your medical team must also give thought to the benefits and drawbacks of treatment, to quality-of-life issues, and to making the decisions that make the most sense. You and they will want to weigh the chance that treatment might be successful against the possible side effects, the time spent in treatment, and the possible limitations on your quality of life.

Your doctor may discover the metastasis during a routine checkup, although sometimes a patient will experience symptoms. It might be bone pain, abdominal discomfort, severe headache, or tingling in the legs. (The latter may occur if a metastasis is pressing on nerves in the spine.) Perhaps weight has been lost without changing exercise or diet habits. One might develop a cough or abdominal pain, or experience hematuria (blood in the urine) or other symptoms of bladder irritation.

Any of these symptoms should send you to the phone to make an appointment with your doctors to figure out whether something sinister is beginning to occur. As you read this you might be thinking that if the cancer is so advanced – if it has spread to the lungs or bones – what's the point of treating symptoms like tingling in your legs or vague abdominal pain?

The point is that even though the cancer has advanced and metastasized, you are likely to live for an extensive period of time – months or years – and it makes good sense to make sure that you are able to live that time comfortably and as fully as possible. If you allow symptoms to go untreated, your ability to participate in everyday life with your family and friends may be greatly diminished, and the time you have left with them may be cut short.

On the other hand, *occasionally* a specialist may decide to watch and wait. For example, when a change is seen on an x-ray but there are no symptoms. Or when a patient is unwell from other medical problems or is just keen to avoid treatment at that time. In such situations, sometimes the decision will be made to observe closely and start treatment when symptoms occur.

What kind of treatment can one expect if the cancer metastasizes?

Surgery to remove the bladder is occasionally a possibility if the only site of recurrence is the bladder and surrounding tissues. It usually doesn't make sense to operate if the cancer has spread to distant sites.

Sometimes radiotherapy will be used to reduce the symptoms of recurrence in the bladder if the recurrence is too extensive to permit surgery or if distant metastases have also occurred.

Chemotherapy is usually used if the cancer has spread widely or to distant sites, and radiotherapy is sometimes used for an isolated metastasis (for example, to the brain or to a bone). A palliative care specialist may be brought in for consultation on how to reduce your pain or make you more comfortable as your disease progresses. And your doctors may talk with you about participating in a clinical trial. (We'll talk about clinical trials later in this chapter.)

For the most part you can expect to remain at home, with any treatment taking place on an outpatient basis. There are exceptions. You might require a short hospital stay to manage a particular symptom, such as resistant pain or a bowel obstruction, but the goal is to have you at home, with your family, participating in as much of life as possible.

CHEMOTHERAPY

As mentioned in the previous chapter, current practice is to blend chemotherapy drugs in order to get a head start in treating the cancer before it becomes too extensive. The goal is increased effectiveness in fighting advanced bladder cancer. This practice has often resulted in a longer and more comfortable lifespan for many bladder-cancer patients and has made it possible to offer increased hope.

A quick review: Chemotherapy is a term that refers to drugs that fight cancer, usually by causing cancer cells to die or causing the process of their growth to stop. It is often a liquid medicine given by injection into the vein. Sometimes it can be administered as a tablet. Chemotherapy treatment is usually provided on an outpatient basis, although certain drugs, such as cisplatin, may be given during a short in-patient stay.

Chemotherapy treatments – which drugs are given and how often – vary from person to person, depending on the stage of disease, the patient's age and overall health, and many other factors. Usually you will receive the drugs intravenously (by needle into the vein), and each treatment will take from one to several hours. You may receive several treatments over the course of a month, and treatments may be given for up to six months or occasionally a bit longer. (More information about chemotherapy is available in Chapter 5, including a detailed discussion of side effects and potential benefits.)

Chemotherapy has many uses. It is given to reduce or eliminate cancer cells present in your body, as well as to prevent existing cancer cells from growing and flourishing. Chemotherapy can inhibit and sometimes prevent the formation of new cancer cells. It can shrink tumors so that they are safely operable. When chemotherapy is used to stop bladder cancer from coming back after treatment by cystectomy or radiotherapy, it is called adjuvant therapy. Chemotherapy is not

Catheter placed in vein

Port placed under skin

Chemotherapy can be given through a surgically implanted port. The "tail" of the port is positioned in a vein so that the chemotherapy drugs go directly into the bloodstream. Only a portion of the "head" of the port (where the chemotherapy is injected) is accessible outside the body. The port remains in the body until treatment comes to an end.

yet able to cure all cancer, but it has certainly opened the door for many people to enjoy many months of extended life.

Again, a reminder: Chemotherapy is powerful medicine. In addition to causing damage to cancerous cells, it can damage cells in the bone marrow that produce blood. This means that your blood count may be lower than usual. A shortage of white blood cells can leave you vulnerable to infections. A low platelet count may lead to bruising or even extensive bleeding from minor cuts and scrapes. Low red blood cell counts leave you feeling fatigued or exhausted (a condition called anemia).

These side effects usually go away after the treatment is stopped. Temporary symptoms such as nausea and vomiting can be controlled to some extent by drugs, while other, more permanent side effects can occur, such as infertility or premature menopause.

DEVELOPMENTS IN THE USE OF CHEMOTHERAPY

There are many chemotherapy drugs or agents, and it has been known for 50 years that some of these can cause advanced or metastatic bladder cancer to shrink or even disappear. The problem is that sometimes the cancer will recover and start to grow again.

Although many anti-cancer or chemotherapy drugs have been shown to work against advanced or metastatic bladder cancer, the list in "routine" use today is somewhat smaller. Before mentioning details of the different drugs, it is worth mentioning that a series of clinical trials (see page 111 for a discussion of clinical trials) has shown that combinations of chemotherapy drugs administered together are *usually* more effective than the use of single drugs. For many years, a combination of four chemotherapy agents (methotrexate, vinblastine, Adriamycin, and cisplatin), the so-called MVAC regimen or treatment, has been used as a standard chemotherapy for advanced bladder cancer. Some years ago, a trial showed that MVAC gave higher shrinkage rates and longer survival than cisplatin alone and that it was also superior to a regimen that combined three drugs (cyclophosphamide, Adriamycin, and cisplatin).

The problem was that it was really quite toxic, with side effects that included nausea, vomiting, a sore mouth, risk of infection, and occasionally problems with cardiac (heart) function. Despite the problems, around 60 percent to 70 percent of patients experienced shrinkage of their metastatic bladder cancers in response to this treatment,

GC vs. MVAC
Overall Survival

A comparison of two chemotherapy regimens routinely used for bladder cancer shows that the survival rates are similar.

and there were patients who survived in good health for several years after such treatment (without recurrence).

Investigators with an interest in bladder cancer have collaborated with scientists to try to find less toxic and more effective drugs than the three-drug regimen. Between 1985 and the present time, several new drugs were identified, including ifosfamide, paclitaxel, docetaxel, and gemcitabine. In a series of clinical trials, each of these drugs showed some activity against advanced bladder cancer. The two that have been most frequently incorporated into modern treatment approaches are paclitaxel and gemcitabine. As single drugs, each has been shown to shrink cancers that have previously received chemotherapy (and have recurred), and they have both been shown to be active against previously untreated cancers.

Today, one of the new standards of chemotherapy for bladder cancer is a combination of gemcitabine and cisplatin. This combination has been shown to cause tumor shrinkage in around 60 percent to 65 percent of cancers and to sustain survival to an extent similar to that of the MVAC regimen. In fact, a trial conducted by the Eli Lilly Corporation (the company that makes gemcitabine), with participation by cancer specialists around the world, specifically examined the combination of gemcitabine-cisplatin in comparison with the MVAC regimen. The proportion of patients surviving in each treatment group was very similar, but the gemcitabine-cisplatin combination was much less toxic than MVAC. As a result, many cancer specialists now view gemcitabine-cisplatin as a new standard of care for patients with metastatic disease. It should be emphasized that a similar randomized clinical trial has not been completed for patients who need neo-adjuvant or adjuvant chemotherapy, and thus the standard in that case remains the MVAC regimen.

Not resting on their laurels, the clinical research community has moved forward and is now testing a new combination that adds paclitaxel, another active drug mentioned above, to the gemcitabine-cisplatin regimen. A three-drug combination (gemcitabine-cisplatin-paclitaxel) has been compared to the two-drug standard, to see whether this produces better cancer shrinkage and improved survival. In June 2007, the first report of this trial was made public. It indicated that the three-drug combination offered no significant benefit compared to gemcitabine-cisplatin and was associated with more side effects.

Another new agent, pemetrexed, also targets the division and reproduction of cancer cells, and has a relatively gentle profile with regard to side effects. It is being tested in patients who have already been treated with gemcitabine and cisplatin to see whether it will cause tumor shrinkage. Early reports are promising, but its true usefulness is not yet known, and it has not yet been assessed by the Food and Drug Administration, which must give formal approval for its use in the treatment of bladder cancer.

In addition to the use of chemotherapy, another class of anti-cancer agents, the so-called growth inhibitors or targeted agents, is being tested in patients with advanced bladder cancer. It is known that proteins located on the surface of cancer cells can control the rate of DNA production and division and stimulate cancer-cell growth. An example is the epidermal growth factor receptor (EGFR), which sits on the surface of some bladder-cancer cells and helps to control the rate at which they grow and divide. Inhibitors of the function of EGFR (and of the genes that control its production) have been developed and are known to slow or stop the growth of some cancer cells.

For example, the agent Herceptin (generic name: trastuzumab) has shown anti-cancer activity in breast cancer, another type of malignancy in which EGFR plays an important role. Trials have been completed in which EGFR inhibitors such as Herceptin have been combined with chemotherapy, and preliminary analysis has suggested the possibility that the combination of Herceptin and chemotherapy may improve results. This is being tested in further clinical trials, to make certain whether this is a true advance and also to discover whether there are "hidden" costs (such as unexpected side effects).

Most recently, preliminary data suggest that a new class of anticancer agents, the tyrosine kinase inhibitors, may also be effective against bladder cancer. For example, the agent sunitinib (brand name: Sutent) has been shown to shrink bladder cancers. This agent helps to inhibit angiogenesis (the formation of tumor-supporting blood vessels) by interacting against a system of enzymes (tyrosine kinases) within the cancer cells that stimulate cancer growth and blood-vessel production. More information will be required before these drugs become a standard of care, and many clinical trials are testing this concept.

CLINICAL TRIALS

A clinical trial is a research study designed to test how well a new drug, therapy, device, or treatment works for people. It's an experimental research process conducted according to strictly regulated scientific and ethical principles that require people who participate in these trials to receive close medical supervision. A clinical trial can *only* be conducted if the patient has been given detailed information about the trial, both written and verbal, and has been given the opportunity to ask questions about benefits and drawbacks to participation. In addition, all clinical trials are reviewed independently by institutional review boards (IRBs), which consider the ethics of the study, the safety for patients, and whether the research is actually worth doing. The protection of your privacy is also an issue that an IRB will oversee, so that information about you is not disclosed inappropriately.

A clinical trial may include fewer than 100 people monitored at just one or two locations, or it can involve thousands of people monitored by many doctors, nurses, data collectors, and other researchers at diverse locations such as doctors' offices, hospitals, clinics, or medical centers.

Clinical trials are sponsored by government agencies such as the National Cancer Institute, along with medical institutions, individual

SOME BENEFITS AND RISKS OF
PARTICIPATION IN A CLINICAL TRIAL

POSSIBLE BENEFITS:

- During a trial you will receive thorough medical monitoring and attention from doctors and other health professionals
- If your cancer is resistant to treatment or has recurred, clinical trials offer another treatment option
- You will receive high-quality cancer care, and if you are in a test group for a new protocol, you may be among the first to benefit from a new treatment that has the potential to be highly effective
- You have the opportunity to help other cancer patients by contributing to the improvement of cancer treatment
- Your participation in a trial may enable you to feel positive and proactive about your treatment plan

POSSIBLE RISKS:

- Your health insurance may not cover all your costs
- The monitoring requirements of the clinical trial may demand more of your time than a non-trial treatment would
- The new treatment being tested may not prove as effective as standard care
- There may be increased or unexpected side effects
- The treatment you receive, whether it is a standard-of-care treatment or a new treatment being tested, may not work for you

doctors or other medical personnel, medical foundations, and drug companies or companies that manufacture diagnostic testing equipment.

You may be alarmed if your doctor suggests the possibility of participating in a clinical trial. Does it mean that you have no hope? What should you do? How should you respond?

It's important not to dismiss the idea out of hand. The words *experimental, research,* and *human volunteer* can be upsetting, particularly at a time when you are dealing with the emotional issues surrounding a diagnosis of advanced cancer. But treatments in clinical trials can often be highly beneficial to those who volunteer. You and your loved ones should talk with your medical team members about the kind of clinical trial they are recommending and why it may benefit you. In fact, several studies have shown that patients participating in clinical trials have better outcomes than those found in the community at large. However, this also may be due to the types of patients who agree to participate in trials.

Does referral to a clinical trial mean that there is no hope of your surviving this illness? Not at all! There is always hope of survival, and any doctor can tell you about people who have responded positively to treatment and not only survived, but thrived. Being in a clinical trial doesn't mean that you won't continue to receive medical treatment; you will, and since it's a voluntary process, you have the right to stop participating in the trial at any time.

As with any aspect of your treatment plan, you make the decision about whether to proceed. Don't feel pressured to participate in a trial if it doesn't feel right for you, but do give it objective thought and consideration.

How do you begin thinking through the decision on whether to participate in a trial?

Probably the first question that comes to your mind is whether clinical trials are safe. Scientists and medical investigators work hard to ensure that they are as safe as possible. The medical community and the U.S. Department of Health and Human Services have put rules in place ensuring that every clinical trial is highly regulated and reviewed by health-care professionals, who determine that the trial is designed and conducted in compliance with federal regulations governing research on human volunteers. Everything about the trial, from the doctors involved to the people who volunteer and the treatment being tested, is subject to strict review and monitoring. However, it is important to understand that some clinical trials *do* carry increased risks.

As with any treatment, you'll want to ask about possible risks, benefits, side effects, how the treatment works, and what results doctors expect from the study. You'll want to know who is conducting the clinical trial and what kind of oversight is in place. Also ask what is expected of you. Where will you go for the treatments? How often will you go? Are there more tests or office visits than you might have with standard treatment? Who administers the treatments and how are the results measured? Do you have to report regularly to those running the trial? Who pays for it all? Will there be extra costs to you as a result of your participation? Will the team conducting the trial (or the doctors involved) stand to benefit personally from the results of the trial or its conduct?

TYPES OF CLINICAL TRIALS

There are many kinds of clinical trials. Some test *prevention,* such as whether vitamin C prevents colds. Some test whether particular *screening* tests, such as mammograms for breast cancer, are effective. The clinical trials your team is likely to mention are *treatment* trials, whereby a new drug, a new treatment, or even a new way of applying a standard treatment, will be examined and tested.

Each treatment trial will have a very detailed and specific plan called a protocol. Think of it as a recipe or instructions that describe what will be done in the trial, why the trial is necessary, who is eligible to participate, and how it will be conducted. Any doctor or researcher who takes part in the trial uses this protocol to ensure consistent results and to make sure that the new drug or treatment is given properly and with maximum safety.

Within treatment trials, there are four categories, or phases. You'll want to ask the members of your medical team which phase of clinical trial they are recommending to you and find out specific details such as the number of people involved, where the testing is being done, what benefits/drawbacks are expected for you personally, and how long the trial is expected to last.

Phase I trials study how to administer a new drug or treatment and how much of the drug or treatment can be safely tolerated. The drugs or treatment in a Phase I trial have been extensively tested in a lab and in animal studies, but not in humans. If a drug is being tested, researchers may start by giving a very low dose of the drug to those participating in the trial, then increase it gradually to determine when side effects appear and what dosage is tolerable, yet effective. Phase I trials usually enroll a small number of people at a limited number of locations. In general, they are the least likely to be of direct personal benefit to a patient, as the drugs are less well known, but occasionally they can lead to significant tumor shrinkage with side effects well within the tolerable range.

Phase II trials take the studies a step further. From the Phase I results, researchers know what dosage to give with a good margin of safely – now they are ready to test whether the drug really works as well as anticipated. They carefully monitor patients in the study for side effects and observe closely how the drug affects the cancer. A Phase II study usually targets a particular disease or type of cancer and includes fewer than 100 people.

Phase III trials involve large groups of people across a broad geographical area. A random process determines which individuals will receive the drug being tested and which ones will receive standard treatment. The idea is to compare accurately whether the new treatment is better than the old treatment and whether there are different patterns of side effects and survival. The results are monitored closely, and if one treatment is observed to be significantly more effective than the other, the trial is stopped. Sometimes a phase III trial will show that the new treatment actually is not better than the standard, in which case the new treatment is usually "dropped" from our list. The reason to "randomize" the study, choosing patients randomly for the new and standard treatments, is to avoid introducing biases into the study. For example, without randomization, there might be an inadvertent tendency to choose the younger and stronger patients for the new agent and older patients with other medical problems for the established treatment. This might make the new treatment appear to be better than the established treatment when, in fact, the differences were due only to the type of patient receiving each type of treatment.

Without randomization, there might be an inadvertent tendency to choose the younger and stronger patients for the new agent and older patients with other medical problems for the established treatment.

Phase IV trials typically take place after the drug or treatment has been approved for standard use. The trial may include up to several thousand people whose medical progress is monitored while they're receiving the drug or treatment. Results are logged to determine how well the drug or treatment is performing in the "real world" (i.e., in a series of doctors' offices and clinics rather than in the setting of a specific clinical comparison trial).

Many trials, particularly Phase III trials, bring together an independent committee of medical professionals, patient advocates, and statistical researchers in a body known as a Data and Safety Monitoring Board (DSMB). The DSMB oversees the trial to ensure that there is no unexpected pattern of serious side effects, that tumor responses are occurring with a reasonable frequency, and that patient welfare is protected. Of course, as previously mentioned, clinical trials cannot occur without approval from an independent or institutional review board (IRB), which reviews the nature, risks, and benefits involved.

Before you are enrolled in a clinical trial, you'll need to meet the eligibility requirements spelled out in the protocol. Eligibility requirements help researchers make sure that results are consistent and that your participation in the trial won't make your condition worse. What kinds of criteria constitute eligibility requirements? Researchers may want people within a specified age range who are a specific sex and

QUESTIONS TO ASK ABOUT CLINICAL TRIALS

- What is the purpose of the trial study and who sponsors it?
- How long will it last?
- Who is monitoring the study? What results are expected?
- How will my safety as a participant be ensured?
- What do I have to do if I participate?
- What procedures or tests are required?
- What are the risks and benefits to me?
- What side effects might I experience?
- What costs will I have to pay? How much will those expenses be? What will my insurance cover?
- What other options do I have regarding my treatment?
- What about new medications? Will I be able to take my regular medications?
- Who will be my doctor? Who is in charge of my care?
- Where will the study take place? Do I have to travel, and if so, who pays?
- Will the study affect my daily life? How?
- Can I drop out at any time?
- Compared to standard care, will there be extra costs or extra risks?
- Do the physicians involved in the trial have any conflict of interest? Do they receive payment for conducting the trial? Are they shareholders in the pharmaceutical company that provides the drug?

who share particular characteristics pertaining to their medical situation and current health. For example, the clinical trial that your doctor recommends to you may be for men between the ages of 60 and 85, who have bladder cancer of a particular type and stage, and who have never previously received chemotherapy.

To help you sort through your questions and concerns is a document called an *informed consent.* This form, which you sign, states that you agree to be in the clinical trial. It includes a disclosure statement from the researcher describing the protocol, who is conducting the trial, what tests will be made and how, the possible risks and the possible benefits to you, and what side effects are anticipated. Informed consent gives you information you need to make a decision about participating in a clinical trial.

Signing an informed consent form does not mean that you are legally bound in any way to remain in the clinical trial. You may drop out at any time. Before the trial starts, after it's under way, during the follow-up period – anytime.

INSTITUTIONS CONDUCTING CLINICAL TRIALS

Recent clinical trials on bladder-cancer treatments (as of July 2007) have taken place or are in progress at the following locations:

- Cleveland Clinic Taussig Cancer Institute, http://cms.clevelandclinic.org/cancer
- Memorial Sloan-Kettering Cancer Center, New York, New York, www.mskcc.org
- M.D. Anderson Cancer Center, Houston, Texas (University of Texas), http://mdanderson.org
- University of Michigan Comprehensive Cancer Center, Ann Arbor, Michigan, www.cancer.med.umich.edu
- University of California, San Francisco, San Francisco, California, http://medschool.ucsf.edu/research
- Dana-Farber/Harvard Cancer Center, Boston, Massachusetts, www.dfhcc.harvard.edu

A reputable place to start looking for current information on cancer centers pursuing clinical trials is the National Cancer Institute's comprehensive clinical trial center (http://cancercenters.cancer.gov). You'll find information there about the cancer centers conducting clinical trials along with links to their websites. (Also see page 152.)

Informed consent doesn't end once the trial has begun. Researchers are obligated to tell you if they find new side effects, benefits, or risks to participating in the study.

WHO PAYS?

Let's say you've decided to participate in a Phase III clinical trial in which a new drug is being tested by a research team. Who pays for it all?

Your usual care costs – those you would incur whether you are enrolled in a trial or not – are usually covered by your insurance plan or Medicare.

It is the extra care costs that are incurred by your participation in a clinical trial that may not be covered. Often if a drug is being tested, it will be provided to you free of charge. But you may have a side effect, such as nausea, and require an anti-nausea prescription. Your insurance company may view this as an extra care cost. The clinical trial may or may not pay for the anti-nausea drugs or other office visits or tests specifically required as part of your being in the trial. Sometimes federal funding or grant programs help pay the costs; sometimes they don't.

If neither the trial nor federal programs cover the cost, it means that you or your insurance company will be expected to pay.

Sadly, your insurance company may or may not agree to pay costs for expenses associated with the clinical trials. Some insurance companies consider such treatment "experimental" and as such, refuse to pay. **Before you agree to participate in a study, make sure that you talk to your insurance company and determine what your plan covers.** Some states have passed legislation requiring insurance companies to cover the costs to patients of clinical trials. At the time this book went to print, Ohio was not one of them. In Ohio, only state employees in the Ohio Med insurance plan have coverage guaranteed by law for certain limited types of clinical trials. Federal health insurance, for the most part, covers clinical trials. Medicare does, for example, and so does health insurance through the Department of Veteran Affairs and the Department of Defense. Things change, however, and you should double-check your coverage before going ahead with a clinical trial.

If your insurance company doesn't cover clinical trial expenses and you want to participate, have someone from your medical team or the clinical trial team contact a representative from your insurance company. Sometimes after claims representatives review the clinical trial protocol, they will approve payment. Also, the National Cancer Institute is working with many health-insurance and managed-care providers to find answers to the question of how to provide coverage for clinical trial participation.

The National Coalition for Cancer Survivorship offers a publication titled *What Cancer Survivors Need to Know About Health Insurance* that helps walk you through the financial maze. You may order the publication at the organization's website (http://www.canceradvocacy.org/resources/publications) or call 1-877-622-7937 to request a copy. The National Cancer Institute's Facing Forward: Life After Cancer Treatments includes a section on insurance issues. It's available at www.cancer.gov or you can order it by calling 1-800-422-6237 (1-800-4-CANCER).

You'll find an extensive list of resources, websites, and helpful publications that deal with a wide range of subjects, including insurance and financial assistance, in Appendix B at the back of this book.

After a clinical trial is over, the results are often published in medical magazines or scientific journals. Once a new drug or treatment has been deemed effective and safe, it becomes standard practice; this means that doctors accept and use the drug or treatment while providing everyday medical care.

The National Library of Medicine has links to the results of many clinical trials at http://www.nlm.nih.gov. ◆

Chapter 7

When Things Don't Work Out

End-of-life decisions are difficult, painful, and heartbreaking. They raise issues we don't want to face, either for ourselves or with someone we love.

Yet at times, despite aggressive and thorough care, there are no further drugs or therapies or surgeries or clinical trials with curative possibilities, and the only option one's medical team has is to recommend hospice care.

The goal of hospice care is not to cure disease; its goal is to provide palliative care – comfort, pain relief, and support – for those facing end-of-life choices. Hospice care addresses quality of life. It involves a team approach similar to the medical team model. Hospice providers offer palliative care specific to those facing an end-of-life diagnosis and their families.

Hospice care doesn't mean that one won't take any more medications or that there may not be some continuing therapies to help with symptoms and quality of life. In the case of advanced bladder cancer, it means that one's medical team has determined that further medical strategies are not likely to cure one's bladder cancer and are not likely to prolong life. Death is the likely outcome, and the emphasis of treatment will change to focus on control of symptoms.

Death. It's such a hard word. Such a scary concept.

The questions pile up in one's mind. Will there be a lot of pain or indignity? What about being physically able to enjoy the rest of life? How to take care of the overwhelming, ongoing business of life?

What about a funeral? What about family? Whom to tell? How to deal with the outpouring of sympathy and questions from family, friends, church members, co-workers? What about cost?

And the emotions pile up in one's heart. The reality of missing so much in the rest of life. The anger and grief about "Why me, why now?" The last time to savor spring's gentle bloom or a grandchild's birthday. Coming to terms with the inevitability of death. The goodbyes.

Those are the sorts of issues – practical, medical, personal, emotional – that a hospice-care team can help with. Let's look at how this process works through a series of questions and answers.

QUESTIONS AND ANSWERS

What is the difference between palliative care and hospice?

Palliative care is a broad term that describes a supportive approach for anyone dealing with a serious or life-threatening illness. Someone who has AIDS, for example, may benefit from palliative care. Palliative care focuses not on curing one's medical situation, but on providing comfort and relief from suffering during or after treatment. Most hospitals have a palliative care team that is separate from hospice. We should not forget that sometimes the palliative care team will help with symptom control for a patient on treatment who may still recover from the cancer.

Hospice is a specific, defined type of compassionate palliative care offered to those facing an end-of-life diagnosis. There are private hospice organizations, both for-profit and nonprofit; in some cases, hospitals have an in-house hospice team. Hospice care can be administered at one's home or in a medical setting such as a hospital or nursing home.

At Cleveland Clinic, Taussig Cancer Institute's Harry R. Horvitz Center for Palliative Medicine and Cleveland Clinic Health Care Ventures, Inc., are among the available options for palliative care or hospice services.

Why all the talk about pain management?
Other than my back starting to ache now and then,
I'm doing okay.

A new or persistent pain, whether a nagging backache or a shooting pain, can signal that one's cancer has changed or grown in some way. Doctors depend on patients to describe any pain, however intermittent or insignificant, so that they can better treat not only the disease, but any affiliated pain as well.

For example, a tender, aching pain in the upper back or shoulder *may* indicate that cancer has moved into the chest cavity or bones. One might feel a squeezing cramp in the abdomen or a shooting pain that feels like an electrical current. However, it is also important to remember that the presence of a new pain doesn't necessarily mean that cancer is active at that site, as pain can be due to many other factors, such as infection or inflammation.

Each of these types of pain tells doctors something different and requires a different combination of drugs and therapies to help them minimize discomfort while they're managing the progression of the disease.

Some people resist telling their doctor about pain because they think that "pain management" involves using drugs such as morphine that leave one pain-free but occasionally in a drowsy fog, and they don't want to spend their days "doped up." Some people simply fear the possibility of addiction, even if they are dying.

Because of the many options available today for pain control, these problems usually don't occur, although the first few days of pain medication (before the optimal dose is found) may be associated with some drowsiness or nausea.

There may be circumstances when narcotic drugs such as morphine are the best option for pain relief. But usually doctors can put together a combination of non-narcotic anti-inflammatory or nonsteroidal anti-inflammatory drugs (such as ibuprofen) that will do the trick while leaving patients alert and able to participate in some of the things they love to do, whether sewing or baking apple pie or even golfing.

There can be side effects from these drugs, such as nausea, shortness of breath, or itching, although most are either temporary or can be controlled with other drugs.

That's not to say that one's days will be a constant round of taking pills and more pills. Some medications are easily absorbed through the skin from a patch or a suppository. Other medications can be injected at regular intervals or even dispensed through a pump (usually implanted under the skin).

And not all pain relief involves drugs. Radiation therapy can relieve some types of bone pain, and doctors can surgically block a nerve's pathway, interrupting the transmission of pain signals to the brain. Acupuncture or electronic nerve stimulation are other ways of managing pain.

Years ago, doctors held off prescribing drugs for pain until the pain was unrelenting. Those days are long gone, and doctors today subscribe to the theory that no one's life should be interrupted by severe pain of any sort. With all the options available for pain management these days, most of them nonintrusive and without significant side effects, there's no reason for one to endure even minimal pain.

I'm feeling well and am still active and involved in my life, even though my doctor told me that I probably only have a year or so to live. Why did she recommend hospice care already?

A medical team is likely to suggest hospice care when there are no drugs or therapies left that are likely to cure one's disease or significantly prolong one's life and when emotional or spiritual comfort and care are needed. Most doctors recommend that patients should begin thinking about hospice when an end-of-life diagnosis has been made, so that they can begin discussing and making decisions about their care and wishes.

Hospice offers an interdisciplinary approach that extends past medical services to embrace and coordinate professional services from many disciplines. A hospice team typically includes one's personal doctor, a hospice physician, nurses, home health aides, social workers, clergy, counselors, other therapists as needed, and a core of trained volunteers.

The hospice team coordinates all aspects of one's care: medical needs, medications, pain, help at home, bereavement counseling, help in a hospital or nursing-home setting, and support for emotional, psychosocial, and spiritual aspects of dying. The hospice team also supports one's family and loved ones.

How do I get into a hospice program?
Where do I find one?

Anyone can call a hospice provider and ask for help, although in most cases, a referral is made from a doctor. In either case, one's doctor must certify eligibility for hospice services. Eligibility generally means that one has been diagnosed with a terminal illness or condition with a life expectancy measured in months rather than years.

Your doctor, senior center, or hospital can probably provide a list of local hospice programs. The National Hospice and Palliative Care Organization also provides help through its website at www.nhpco.org and by phone at 1-800-658-8898. Medline Plus has a state-by-state list of providers at http://medlineplus.gov. In Ohio, referrals are available through www.hospiceohio.org.

Choosing hospice does not mean giving up hope. It does mean choosing a strategy to maximize one's quality of life while stabilizing one's medical condition and getting practical help in planning a comfortable, supported, and pain-free end of life. Sometimes facing the prospect of death overpowers the remaining gifts that life has to offer. Hospice can ease some of the burdens – financial, medical, and emotional – and offer opportunities to savor each sunrise, each crisp apple or juicy peach, each hug from a friend or loved one, and the gifts of laughter and love and memories.

Who pays for hospice? My insurance? Me?

Medicare and most private insurance companies pay for hospice expenses. Most hospices are certified by Medicare, and most people who use hospice are over 65, the age of eligibility for Medicare. The Medicare Hospice Benefit, available to those with Part A Medicare, pays for virtually every cost associated with hospice care, from medications to counseling services.

> Choosing hospice does not mean giving up hope. It does mean choosing a strategy to maximize one's quality of life while stabilizing one's medical condition and getting practical help in planning a comfortable, supported, and pain-free end of life.

Most insurance companies have provisions for paying for hospice benefits for those under the age of 65. However, hospice programs certified by Medicare are required to provide a specific set of core services to anyone needing hospice care regardless of insurance.

Hospice benefits don't cover any ongoing medications or therapies prescribed for cure rather than comfort.

What is hospice? A place?

It can be. Some hospice providers have private care facilities, but in most cases, hospice is provided in one's home, in the hospital, or in a nursing home. Hospice is a type of service, not a place.

What if I don't like hospice? Am I stuck?

No. One can leave hospice at any time and reinstate regular health-care benefits and care. Conversely, one can go back to hospice at any time, provided that one remains eligible. Hospice benefits can remain in place indefinitely, although one must periodically be re-certified as eligible.

There are lots of hospice programs around. How do I know which one is best?

Asking for recommendations from health-care professionals, nursing homes, clergy, senior centers, or trustworthy people who have used hospice services in the past is a good place to start. The National Hospice and Palliative Care Organization (NHPCO) maintains a helpline at 800-658-8898 (and a website at www.nhpco.org) that can provide assistance as well. NHPCO has a comprehensive tool called "Standards and Practices for Hospice Programs" that is complex but offers detailed information on how hospice programs should be structured and should handle specific concerns.

What should I ask a hospice agency?

Before making a choice, interview the hospice agency. Below are some questions to get you started.

- What services are provided?
- How involved will my doctor be in my care?
- What support services are available to me and my family, and how do we take advantage of them?
- How many volunteers do you have? What kind of training do they get? What sort of services are your volunteers involved in?
- What happens if something is needed outside normal business hours?
- Is your program certified by Medicare?
- What if in-patient care is needed? How is it handled?
- What about pain? What do you do for comfort?

- Who will be on my interdisciplinary team? How many families does it care for at once? How often will the nurse visit?
- Do you ask families to complete a satisfaction survey, and if so, may I see the results?
- Are you accredited by any professional organizations? Do they perform periodic inspections, and if so, may I see the results?
- What happens if I can't stay in my home because of increasing care needs?
- Who pays for this, and is it mostly covered by insurance?

Do I have to sign anything like a living will?

Hospice providers believe in death with dignity, and they affirm death as a natural, normal process. As such, hospice respects patients' goals, preferences, and choices as long as those choices neither prolong life through active anti-cancer therapy nor hasten death. In most cases, those receiving hospice care choose to sign *advance directives*, documents designed to tell family members and medical professionals what kind of care should be provided if and when the patient is no longer able to make such decisions.

For example, a *living will* is a legal document that describes what kind of life-sustaining medical treatments you want, if any. A *durable power of health care* lets you choose the person you want to make health-care decisions for you, if necessary. A Do Not Resuscitate (DNR) document instructs medical professionals not to perform cardio-pulmonary resuscitation (CPR) or other life-saving efforts if you stop breathing or your heart stops. These documents are legal in most states, and your doctor's office or hospice team can tell you where to get forms. Online forms and a description of advance directives are available through the NHPCO site (www.nhpco.org), which links to www.caringinfo.org/AdvanceDirectives. Information can also be found at the AARP site (www.aarp.org/research/legal/advancedirect).

In keeping with the hospice philosophy "neither hasten nor postpone death," many hospice organizations ask for a signed DNR; they may or may not require other advance directives.

WHAT YOU NEED TO KNOW ABOUT LIVING WILLS

- A living will lets you determine *in advance* and *while you are able* what kind of medical care you want if you are *unable* to express your wishes because you are terminally ill or permanently unconscious. (If you are able to tell your doctor what care you want, a living will cannot be invoked.)

- Laws governing living wills vary from state to state. Check with your state government or an attorney to determine what is required.Websites with information on state laws include: http://estate.findlaw.com/estate-planning/living-wills.html and http://www.caringinfo.org. Your living will gives your doctor(s) the authority to allow you to die naturally, without life-sustaining treatment other than that necessary to make you comfortable or to relieve your pain.

- In your living will, you have the choice of *giving* or *not giving* your doctor the authority to withhold food administered through a feeding tube. You decide in advance whether you want your life extended if the time comes when you require such artificial means of life support.

- The law requires your doctor to make every effort to notify your closest relatives if your living will is invoked. Your closest relatives have the right to legally challenge the doctor on whether your medical condition is such that your living will should be invoked, but no one can legally challenge your right to determine for yourself whether you want or do not want your life extended by artificial means.

- A living will can't be enforced if your family, persons holding powers of attorney, physicians, or caregivers don't know about it. Make sure your loved ones and health-care professionals who provide your care (including hospital officials) have a copy of your living will.

- You may revoke your living will at any time simply by informing your doctor of your intent. It's a good idea to ask for any copies of your living will to be returned to you, and you should then destroy the copies.

- Your living will takes precedence over a health-care power of attorney. A living will takes effect when you are permanently unable to express your wishes; a health-care power of attorney designates someone to make health-care decisions for you if you are temporarily unable to do so yourself.

How long does it take for hospice care to start?

In most cases, hospice care starts almost immediately after a referral is made. Typically, a hospice worker will meet with you and your doctor within 48 hours and begin working on a plan of care that includes among many other things an evaluation of the services and medications you or your loved ones might need. Some of the options might include a medication plan or a referral to a grief group or cancer support group.

I don't know whether hospice is right for me. I'm feeling hopeless about what's facing me. Where can I turn for support?

For a careful and candid discussion about your choices and expectations, your own doctor is often a good place to start.

Cleveland Clinic's toll-free Patient Resource Cancer Information Line (1-866-223-8100) is another good option, especially if your doctor is not certain or is reluctant to discuss such matters. Two cancer nurses are available to answer questions and provide resource help from 8:00 a.m. to 4:30 p.m. Monday through Friday. (You don't have to be a Cleveland Clinic patient to call the Cancer Line.)

There are many support groups available for cancer patients and their families and friends. Cleveland Clinic's social work department (1-216-444-6552) or the Cancer Answer Line (1-800-862-7798) can help you find a group that meets your needs, and so can the American Cancer Society (1-800-227-2345 or www.cancer.org). The American Cancer Society website also has public message boards for those who wish to participate.

At the downtown campus at Cleveland Clinic, the Patient Resource Center at Taussig Cancer Institute is open Monday through Friday from 8:00 a.m. to 4:30 p.m. The Resource Center offers brochures about cancer, listings about support groups and resources, and computer terminals for Internet searches.

The National Cancer Institute's Information Service (1-800-422-6237 or 1-800-4-CANCER) can provide help to patients and their families who need to locate programs, services, or resources.

The Visiting Nurse Association of America (www.vnaa.org or 1-888-866-8773) can provide resources for skilled nursing, mental-health care, hospice care, or home health care.

CAREGIVER STRESS

The patient is not the only one who's having a rough time. Sometimes those caring for loved ones with cancer don't pay enough attention to taking care of themselves. They are so focused on the daily responsibilities of providing good care to the person who is ill that they overlook their own need for rest and food and exercise.

How do you know when you've crossed the line from "good care-giving" to "caregiver stress?"

For one thing, maybe you can't go to sleep, or if you do, you are restless. Because you aren't sleeping well, you feel tired and burned-out all the time. That fatigue can lead to being irritable and short on patience. You start to feel like a zombie, doing things by rote and with-out enough attention, or perhaps you resent having to do so much for someone else and feel guilty about feeling resentful. You might eat too much, or not care about eating at all. Maybe you've started to drink a second – or third – glass of wine.

Any or all of the above can be signs that you're not taking enough time to take care of yourself.

You're probably shaking your head and thinking, "I know that. But what can I do to change it? Someone has to be there night and day, giv-ing medication and baths and changing the sheets three times a day."

You're right. Someone does have to be there. But perhaps it doesn't always have to be you. Can you afford to have a home care worker come in for a few hours once a week? If not, is there a friend, relative, or neighbor who might relieve you? If you can't work some-thing out with a paid home care worker or friend, talk to your doctor or social worker. There are options.

Once you have an hour or two for yourself, what do you do? First of all, don't feel guilty about taking a little time for yourself. Think of

CHOOSING A HOME CARE AGENCY

- Here are a few questions to have handy when you're looking for home care for yourself or a loved one.

- Is the agency licensed by the state? Certified by Medicare? Accredited by a national organization such as the Joint Commission on Healthcare Accreditation?

- How long has the agency been providing cancer care? Does the agency provide the services you need or expect you will need? Does the agency own or can it arrange for equipment that you (or home care staff) might need?

- How are home care workers hired, trained, supervised, and monitored? Are they licensed?

- Who bills Medicare and insurance, you or the agency? Who follows up on claims?

- What happens if you need emergency care? What happens if a home care worker doesn't show up? Is there a 24-hour contact available?

- Did the agency explain to you the rights of the patient?

- Do you feel comfortable talking with agency personnel? What if you have a complaint?

- Can the agency provide references from current clients?

it as recharging yourself so that you can go back to your caretaking duties refreshed and alert.

You probably have a long list of errands to do and your first thought may be to fill those free hours by going to the dry cleaner's, the hardware store, or Target. While it's fine to drop off a pair of shoes for repair while you're out and about, do reserve this time to do something *refreshing*.

Go to the library and sit in a quiet corner to read. Get your nails done or have a massage. Go out to lunch or play nine holes of golf with a friend. Go to the gym or recreation center and have a swim and a sauna. You get the idea – do something for YOU.

Even if you can't get away for a short time every day, there are things you can do to ease the daily stress. Buy a yoga DVD to use at home or indulge yourself by watching a favorite television program. If you like to read, why not read a book aloud to the person you are caring for, or pop some corn and watch a movie together? Finding ways to smile and laugh each day makes a big difference, too.

If you are able, join a caregiver's support group. Not only will it help you feel refreshed, but you might learn some great tips about being a caregiver and find some sympathetic shoulders to cry on when the going gets tough. These days, online support groups make it possible to connect with others even when you *can't* get away.

Do be cautious in joining online groups, however. You might want to read the article "How to Find an Online Support Group" at the American Cancer Society's website, www.cancer.org. The ACS has its own online support resources at its Cancer Survivors Network, http://www.acscsn.org.

CARES FOR CAREGIVERS

Olympic gold-medalist and cancer survivor Scott Hamilton learned first-hand how scary cancer can be for both patients and the loved ones responsible for their care, and he decided to do something about it. With Cleveland Clinic Taussig Cancer Institute, he established the Scott Hamilton CARES Initiative (Cancer Alliance for Research, Education and Survivorship) for patients and their families. From this, the 4th Angel mentoring program for caregivers was born.

This national program pairs mentors who have been caregivers with "new" caregivers who need firsthand answers to some very hard questions. Mentors and caregivers meet by phone or through e-mail; all you need to do to be paired with a 4th Angel mentor is to call 1-866-520-3197 or visit www.scottcares.com.

ADVANCED BLADDER CANCER
CASE STUDY: TIM, AGE 70

For four or five months, Tim hadn't been feeling himself. He'd been tired, for one thing. Really tired. He started taking a multivitamin, thinking that he might be low in iron, but it didn't seem to help. He tried fixing himself healthier meals, but half the time he'd scrape most of what he cooked down the disposal. Nothing much tasted good anymore.

Then he started noticing spots of blood in his underwear. He figured he had a kidney problem. Maybe a kidney stone. That would account for the persistent dull ache in his side, too. He bought a jug of cranberry juice but before he could drink it all, the spots of blood became a daily thing and he decided he'd better call his doctor and get things checked out.

"You've lost nine pounds since the last time you were here," the nurse announced after she weighed Tim. "You'd better stop dieting. You're getting a little too skinny."

"I'm not dieting," Tim said. "I don't have much of an appetite these days, that's all."

Dr. L examined Tim, asking a lot of questions about when Tim had noticed the spotting and the ache in his side, and whether he felt any pain in his lower back.

"What do you think is wrong?" Tim asked. The serious look on the doctor's face worried him. Tim had been coming to Dr. L for a long time, maybe 15 years, and the doc usually joked and asked Tim about where he'd been fly-fishing lately. Today Dr. L was all business.

"I think we need to do some tests, Tim. A CT scan, a urinalysis, and a bone scan, for starters."

"A bone scan? That's not good, I know that." Tim buttoned his shirt. "Look, just tell me what you think is going on. I'll only imagine the worst if you don't."

Dr. L explained that while he didn't want to jump to any conclusions before he got the test results, he suspected that Tim was seriously ill.

"The bones in your lower back are tender, your liver is enlarged, you've lost weight, and you've experienced intermittent hematuria, or blood in your urine," said Dr. L. "I suspect either a serious infection or possibly cancer, but we won't know for sure until we get the test results."

As soon as the word was out of Dr. L's mouth, Tim realized that he'd been swallowing worry about cancer ever since the nurse pointed out how much weight he'd lost. Tim knew that unplanned weight loss was a sign of cancer.

When Tim came in for his follow-up appointment after his tests, Dr. L sat behind his desk, papers arranged neatly in a pile in front of him, hands folded. *Not good news,* thought Tim. *If it were good news, he'd at least smile.*

Instead, Dr. L straightened some papers and started talking in a calm, low voice. Each word he spoke added to Tim's fear and worry. Large deposits in the liver. Blood in his urine. Spots of cancer on his rib bones. Bladder cancer that has spread to other parts of his body.

"So what do we do about all this?" asked Tim. "What kind of treatment? There's so much you can do these days for cancer."

"Well, I'm going to refer you to an oncologist at Taussig Cancer Institute for the answer to that question, Tim. We'll work as a team, but for advanced cancer treatment, you need a specialist."

"How soon can I get in?" Now that the diagnosis of cancer was for sure, Tim felt as if he had to do something. Right then. Get the cancer out or start doing something to kill it. He couldn't just sit still and wait for appointments.

"As long as it takes us to cross the street," said Dr. L. "One of the Clinic's oncologists is working out of the Strongsville branch today, and my nurse arranged for her to meet with us this afternoon."

Before the two men left the office, Tim said, "You know, I've been coming here a long time, since before Sadie died. You can be straight with me. How bad is it?"

"That's another question we need to ask the oncologist. Bladder cancer isn't my specialty, and whatever statistics I'd give you are likely to be outdated or flat-out wrong. But I can tell you it's serious, Tim."

Tim nodded. "Okay. Fair enough."

Aggressive Treatment

The oncologist laid it straight out for Tim. "We're going to do an aggressive regimen of chemotherapy with gemcitabine and cisplatin, drugs that have a proven track record against bladder cancer. It's not such a tough regimen, Tim. You'll probably experience mild nausea and tiredness and perhaps tingling in your feet. And there's risk of infection. I can give you some medications to help with the side effects but they won't be alleviated entirely."

Tim nodded. He appreciated the doctor's frankness in explaining what lay ahead of him.

"With this aggressive regiment of Gem-Cis, we have a 40 to 60 percent chance of shrinking the cancer."

"Wow, that's a better cure rate than I expected," said Tim. Dr. L and the oncologist exchanged a somber look. "What was that look about? Is there something you're not telling me? Look, I can handle this if I know what's going on, what to expect. What I can't handle is uncertainty and worry."

"That's fair, Tim, and I'll try to meet your expectations." The doctor cleared her throat. "There is always hope for a cure, but we cannot be sure. At this stage of advanced cancer, Tim, your chances of a permanent cure are less than 10 percent. What you need to keep in mind is that while the chemotherapy may not cure your disease at this point, it may stop any further spread of the disease and hopefully, result in a remission (or tumor shrinkage) that might last for months or even years. Your chances of a remission are about 40 percent."

Tim sat quietly for a moment. The odds weren't as good as he'd hoped. But someone had to be among the 40 percent who had a remission. Tim would do everything possible to make sure he was one of them.

"I can deal with those odds," he said. "It's almost even-steven. You just tell me what I need to do to help myself be one of the 40 percent, and I'll do it."

Tim had a rough time with the chemotherapy, but he refused to give up or lose hope. And indeed, he was one of the lucky ones. He went into remission after his Gem-Cis treatment and for 14 months spent every available moment with his son and two grandchildren.

"These babies are better than chemotherapy," he kept saying. "And fewer side effects, too."

Then, just after his 72nd birthday, Tim felt an ache in his gut. He ignored it for a few days, but when it didn't go away, he went back to see his oncologist, who ordered a round of blood tests, a bone scan, and a CT scan.

Tim knew the news wouldn't be good, and it wasn't. His cancer was back. It was in his liver and bones again.

His doctor told him that it was time to consider two things: a clinical trial and hospice care.

"I don't much care for the idea of being a guinea pig," said Tim. "But if I can help find a better treatment or a cure for this disease, then I'll do it."

His doctor told him that it was time to consider two things: a clinical trial and hospice care.

"I'm going to refer you to a social worker, Tim. She'll help you through the process of deciding about a clinical trial, and she'll get you some information about hospice."

"I'm not ready for hospice," Tim said. "Maybe down the road, when I'm not doing so well . . ."

His doctor said, "I think you should think about it now. I know you're not ready, but it's much easier to get the paperwork done now and get to know the people now that you'll be working with in hospice, before it's a crisis situation. It's hard to let outsiders like hospice caregivers into your family at a private time like this, Tim, but I don't think you'll be sorry. Hospice can make a big difference."

His doctor gave Tim a brochure about a Phase II cancer trial under way at Cleveland Clinic.

"I'll talk to my son. We've already talked about this a little, and he's all for me doing what I can to help the research efforts. He's an optometrist and knows how much research has benefited his field."

"I think you told me that about your son. I hope you'll take part, Tim, but if you don't, that's okay. Clinical trials aren't for everyone. Some people want the reassurance of being treated by their doctor at their hospital. Others get a lift from helping research efforts."

The Cancer Progresses

Tim's cancer progressed more quickly than anyone expected. Within four weeks, the pain in his back and abdomen had returned. Sometimes it was quite intense. He was glad he'd taken his oncologist's advice and let his social worker set up hospice care for him. He just didn't feel like struggling further, and he changed his mind about the clinical trial.

A nurse and hospice social worker came to his house a few days after his appointment with his oncologist. They explained how hospice works and talked about the hospice philosophy of care.

"Our goal is to help create a place of rest and comfort for you and your family," said Nancy, Tim's hospice nurse. "We provide comfort care and make sure your pain and symptoms are under control so you can live your life with as much gusto as possible and even fulfill some of your life wishes. We offer a team approach to meeting your spiritual, physical, and emotional needs. And we try to help you accept the process of dying while embracing life. It's a complex emotional time, one that can bring fear, hope, worry, grief, sadness, joy, anger, and eventually, peace."

The hospice social worker helped Tim put in place a living will and a durable power of health care. Tim didn't want to prolong his life with any breathing machines or feeding tubes, so he talked to his social worker about signing a Do Not Resuscitate (DNR) order.

Tim showed his son the documents and explained that he wanted to die as peacefully and painlessly as possible. It was a sad afternoon, and the two of them shared not only tears but laughter. They looked at old pictures and videotapes, drank Tim's favorite root beer, and ate a whole plate of peanut-butter cookies that Tim's neighbor had brought over.

It wasn't too long before Tim started feeling enough pain that his hospice team suggested a regimen of medications and massage therapy for him. They arranged for a hospital bed and for a home care worker to cook and clean for Tim a few times a week.

"It's amazing what these people do for me, how much they care,"

Tim told his son. "They make this whole thing bearable and manageable, and believe me, sometimes it's just so overpowering that I can't think or function. I wouldn't have known where to turn or what to do without them."

Tim sat quietly for a minute before continuing. "You know, sometimes in the middle of the night hopelessness gets the best of me and I feel so alone in the darkness, so afraid. I mentioned it one time to Nancy when she said the black circles under my eyes looked like bruises. And you know what she did? She gave me a number I can call anytime, day or night, to talk to someone in hospice. I never have called. Maybe because the comfort of knowing I *can* call helps get me through the night."

"Dad, you can always call me, anytime."

"I know, son, but you're dealing with your own emotions about all this. I hate to lean on you too much. I like it that our visits are mostly talk about the kids and what they're doing and everyday things. It makes me feel normal, and that's nice."

Once the symptoms were brought under control, Tim decided to consider the clinical trial again. He was adamant about wanting to participate. Nancy, the oncologist, Tim, and his son sat down to talk about it together. They hashed over whether the regimen of medication and follow-up care would be too much for Tim, and talked about whether the possible side effects might impair the quality of his life.

"Will this be a benefit or a burden, Tim?" asked Nancy. "Is it worth it?"

"You bet it's worth it," said Tim. "It's probably too late for me to benefit from this trial, but you know, maybe someday my son or someone else's son will be diagnosed with bladder cancer. And I'd like to think that if that happens, there will be a new and promising treatment available … and that I helped make that possible."

Tim's son hugged him. "Dad, you are an incredible man."

"If I were so incredible, I would've stopped smoking years ago. The day you were born. But the fact is, I wouldn't want to do this if you hadn't inspired me, son." Tim took a pen and signed the consent forms for the clinical trial. "But I've come to feel that doing this means that my life will be remembered in some small way. As if I'll participate in creating a legacy for future generations, and there will be a breath of my spirit in those who benefit from the research. That's a bit of peace and comfort I didn't expect from all this. And you know, I might be one of the lucky ones and respond to the treatment, right?"

When Tim stopped speaking, there wasn't a dry eye in the room.

COPING WITH GRIEF

Grief is all about loss. It may be your grief about losing the rest of your life to cancer. It may be your loved ones' grief about losing you to cancer. Either way, emotions are varied – from shock, sadness, worry, and guilt to emptiness, anger, or fear – and they come and go with amazing speed.

Maybe you can't concentrate on anything, even something as familiar as writing checks to pay bills. Maybe you wake up a lot at night or have bad dreams. You may not care about cooking meals, let alone eating them. You may cry a lot or feel numb, or experience what seems like unending waves of sadness.

It may not seem like it, but all those emotions and feelings are not only part of the grief process, they're part of the healing process as well.

Here are some things you can do to work through the grief process.

Be with people. Friends, family, loved ones. Let them buoy your spirits and ease a bit of your pain.

Do normal things, even though sometimes you might not feel like it. Go out to dinner with friends. Plant your garden. Clean the house. Get a pet. It's okay to do these things; it doesn't mean you are forgetting your circumstances or betraying the person who is gone.

Follow the three Es:
- Exercise; it lifts your mood.
- Eat right. Your body needs fuel even if you never feel hungry anymore.
- Express yourself. Talk about your emotions and feelings if you can. If you can't, try writing in a journal or talking to yourself while having a good cry. Don't hesitate to talk to your doctor or a therapist.

The Three E's: Exercise, Eat Right, and Express Yourself

Think about joining a support group. Sometimes you feel as if your grief is a burden to your family or friends. In a support group, you can speak freely with those who are experiencing similar losses.

Do good in someone else's name. Sometimes taking action as a tribute to a loved one helps a lot. Run a race for cancer, donate books to a library in your loved one's name, or plant a special rose bush in your garden. Tributes have a way of bringing some peace to the pain of grief.

We are not suggesting that you measure the course of your feelings against an artificial schedule, but if time has passed, say four or five months, and you still feel deep, intense grief or depression – or if you're feeling suicidal at any time – it's probably time to talk to someone, perhaps your doctor or social worker or a good friend, about getting professional help in working through your feelings. ◆

Chapter 8

The Health-Care System

Those who have bladder cancer may have different types of the disease or be in different stages, but they all have one thing in common: Before long, they're buried under a blizzard of paperwork and appointments and things to handle.

There are insurance forms. Applications to clinical trials. Prescription refills. Explanations of benefits from the hospital and insurance companies. Instructions on how to prepare for tests or take medications. Forms at work requesting family leave. Maybe you live a fair distance from the hospital and have to arrange for accommodations when you have appointments or perhaps you need help with child care.

There are insurance forms. Applications to clinical trials. Prescription refills. Explanations of benefits from the hospital and insurance companies. Instructions on how to prepare for tests or take medications.

It's overwhelming, and it comes at a time when you may be feeling least able to deal with such demanding issues.

What do you do? Where do you turn for help?

In most cases, your hospital's social work department is a good place to start. You can ask your doctors or nurses for a referral, or you can call the department directly.

At Cleveland Clinic, for example, social workers at the Taussig Cancer Institute can help you sort through many of the topics we'll talk about in this chapter. They can be a lifeline on days when you don't know where to turn. You can reach the Taussig Cancer Institute's social workers through the toll-free Cancer Hotline at 1-866-223-8100.

INSURANCE MATTERS

The bills and explanations of benefits and notification of payments from insurance companies or Medicare pile up fast when you are undergoing complex cancer treatment, and it's often hard to figure out what has been paid, what hasn't, and how much you owe to the hospital, doctors, or service providers such as imaging centers.

Sometimes it seems as if the insurance statements are so hard to understand, they might as well be written in Latin, doesn't it?

Social workers can help steer you through the paperwork maze and sometimes even act as your advocate in the case of a dispute.

IF YOU DON'T HAVE INSURANCE

Some people don't receive health insurance as an employment benefit and can't afford to buy it on their own. Others may have exceeded their coverage or have only limited insurance that doesn't cover some tests, treatments, medications, or clinical trials. Maybe you aren't eligible for insurance or aren't working for some reason and simply don't have coverage. Even worse, maybe you can't keep working because of your illness.

What happens if you don't have insurance or you've lost it? What can a social worker do to help you?

Depending on your income level, you might be eligible for Medicaid coverage. If you are disabled and collect Social Security, you might be eligible for a Medicare hospitalization plan, regardless of your age.

If you had to leave your job, you might be able to obtain extended benefits through a state plan called COBRA, which lets you pay to maintain your previous insurance coverage for 18 months after leaving your employer.

There are some community resources available, too. Your social worker can guide you through the process of finding and applying for insurance or assistance.

IF INSURANCE WON'T PAY OR YOU'RE TURNED DOWN

Insurance companies can turn you down if you apply for a new policy and have a preexisting condition such as bladder cancer. They can't, however, stop your existing coverage if you are diagnosed with an illness *so long as you keep your premiums paid up.*

Luckily, there is help available for many people who have limited health insurance or none, and your social worker can help you work through the process of applying for it.

For one thing, you can apply for an individual health policy during certain periods of the year designated "Open Enrollment." During these times, you can't be turned down for a preexisting condition. Some insurers or HMOs accept those with preexisting conditions but require a waiting period that can be as long as six months before coverage takes effect.

FINANCIAL ASSISTANCE

Even with some of the above safeguards in place, many people can't afford or aren't eligible for health-insurance coverage and the medical bills start mounting up at a fearsome rate.

Ohio has a plan in place, the Ohio Hospital Care Assurance Program (HCAP), to make sure that people under the federal poverty level who aren't on the Medicaid plan receive free, basic, medically necessary hospital services. Cleveland Clinic goes a step beyond HCAP and gives free hospital services or assistance with financial arrangements for medical care to those without insurance who have income levels up to four times higher than the federal poverty level.

> Ohio has a plan in place, the Ohio Hospital Care Assurance Program (HCAP), to make sure that people under the federal poverty level who aren't on the Medicaid plan receive free, basic, medically necessary hospital services.

GOT QUESTIONS? GET ANSWERS!

One of your medications costs more for one day's dose than your groceries cost for a week and you're not sure you can keep taking it because of the expense. Whom do you talk to? Your doctor? Your oncologist? A nurse? A social worker?

If your questions are of a medical nature, talk to your doctor, physician's assistant, or nurse. If you have family concerns, need emotional or financial resources, or even just want some guidance on talking with your loved ones about your cancer, you can also contact your social worker.

The key to getting answers is *asking questions.* You may feel as if your concerns are insignificant or that there isn't likely to be an easy solution. Or perhaps you don't want to bother your doctor or social worker. Don't feel that way. There are amazing resources out there, but if the members of your team don't know of your concern, they can't help you tap into those resources. And they want to help you. Doctors, nurses, and social workers all want you to be actively involved in your treatment. Communication between you and your team is paramount.

Communication is more than just asking questions. Getting answers that you understand is equally important. If the answer you get from your treatment team isn't clear, whether it is a response to a medical question or a question about insurance coverage, ask for a better explanation.

Prepare for conversations or appointments by writing down your questions or concerns *and* taking notes on the answers. (If you want to listen rather than take notes, bring someone along to act as your recording secretary.)

Many people feel that they lose control of their lives when they are being diagnosed and treated for cancer. By asking questions and learning about your illness, you can help maintain your participation in choices pertaining to your care. Your team can support you in many ways, whether it's helping you find a support group or information about clinical trials, or guiding you through the maze of insurance coverage or medication assistance.

FINANCIAL ASSISTANCE FOR MEDICATIONS

If you don't have prescription drug coverage, some pharmaceutical companies have programs that make the cost of medications more reasonable. Most companies limit the amount of income you can earn and still remain eligible for medication assistance, but the income ceilings are usually much higher than the federal poverty level or the upper limit of Medicaid eligibility.

Don't ever hesitate to inquire about whether the cost of your prescriptions might be covered through an assistance program, especially if you are doing without food or necessities to buy needed medication – or doing without the medication.

Besides medication assistance for those without a prescription plan and who meet income eligibility requirements, there are low-cost prescription plans provided through many of the pharmaceutical companies for seniors enrolled in Medicare and people with disabilities who receive Medicare. Your physician or social worker will be able to advise you about which companies provide such benefits.

> **Don't ever hesitate to inquire about whether the cost of your prescriptions might be covered through an assistance program, especially if you are doing without food or necessities to buy needed medication.**

The programs work in a variety of ways. In some cases, necessary medications are provided directly through the drug company for either a small fee or sometimes no cost at all. More often, you are issued a card, such as the Orange Card or the Together Rx card, that provide discounts on prescriptions or even some services such as dental and vision.

There are dozens of programs with varying criteria that offer hundreds of covered medications. While that's a good thing for you if you need prescription assistance, it can be dizzying to compare the programs and sort out what is covered and how much it will cost you.

Luckily, your social worker can help you find sources of medication assistance and is able to help you decide what program best suits your needs.

SEARCHING FOR AFFORDABLE
MEDICATIONS: A STARTING POINT

If you want to do some research on your own, you can check out eligibility criteria and covered medications by calling a number of organizations toll-free or visiting their websites. Among them are:

- **Needy Meds.** This group lists most major drugs and drug company programs. Some applications are available at the website (www.needymeds.com).

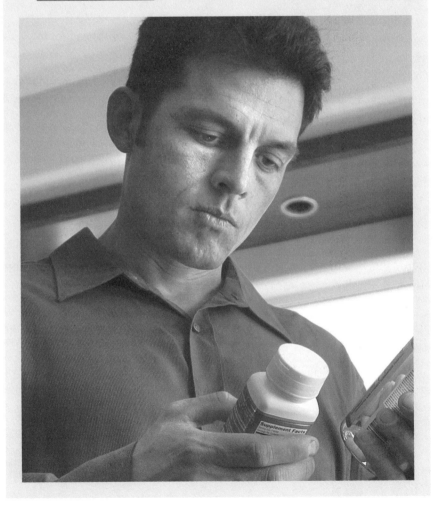

● **RxAssist.** You'll find similar information here, with a comparative chart of most drug-discount programs. (Go to www.rxassist.org or call 1-877-844-8442.)

● **Partners for Prescription Assistance (PPARx.org).** This site is a portal to 475 public and private programs (including more than 180 programs offered by pharmaceutical companies) that help eligible patients obtain free or nearly free medications. (Go to https://www.pparx.org/Intro.php or call the toll-free number: 1-888-477-2669 or 1-888-4PPA-NOW.)

There also are programs sponsored by individual pharmaceutical companies or by consortiums of pharmaceutical companies. This is a sample listing of available programs:

● **LillyMedicareAnswers** is sponsored by Eli Lilly and Company for patients needing medications not covered by Medicare Part D. Applications can be obtained by visiting the website (www.LillyMedicareAnswers.com) or calling 1-877-795-4559 or 1-877-RX-LILLY.

● **Pfizer Sharecard** (www.pfizer.com) is for those age 65 or older or other Medicare enrollees; prescriptions cost $15 for a 30-day supply with a Sharecard.

● **SaveWell,** administered by Medical Mutual of Ohio, offers discounted prescriptions as well as discounted vision and dental care. (Go to www.savewell.com or call 1-877-728-3935 or 1-877-SAVEWELL.)

● **Together Rx Card** is open to seniors and others on Medicare. The program offers discounted prescriptions from seven major pharmaceutical companies. (Go to www.togetherrxaccess.com or call 1-800-444-4106.)

● **Orange Card** is provided through GlaxoSmithKline pharmaceuticals to offer discounts on GSK medications to seniors and others on Medicare. Applications can be obtained from health-care providers or by calling 1-888-672-6436 or 1-888-ORANGE6.

PATIENT SUPPORT AND ADVOCACY

It's hard not to feel like the "little guy" amid all the insurance companies, hospital departments, and government agencies. And sometimes, despite everyone's best efforts, you might feel as if you aren't getting the treatment or attention you deserve.

How do you voice your concerns and worries when it seems as if everyone else is more important or has more clout than you have?

You talk to your social worker, who can act as your advocate. That sounds good, but what does "acting as your advocate" mean?

The word advocate means someone who speaks or acts on your behalf. Someone who takes up your cause, your issues, and who fights for your interests. It means that someone who knows how to get around in the health-care system serves as your voice.

Perhaps your concern is that you feel you need someone to talk to. That you feel alone and adrift and afraid of what is going to happen to you. Your social worker can help you. That's why many hospitals, including Cleveland Clinic, have social work offices right in their cancer centers. Social workers are the first to be called in an emotional crisis and are able to provide immediate counseling as well as help you find resources such as support groups.

If the idea of telling your feelings and problems to a group doesn't appeal to you, some hospitals have something similar to Cleveland Clinic's 4th Angel program, which pairs bladder-cancer patients (or caregivers) with someone of similar age and sex who has gone through bladder-cancer treatment. The two of you can talk privately and confidentially about what it's like to go through treatment and live with cancer.

Perhaps your concerns are more along the lines of whether you should participate in a clinical trial. Or perhaps you feel that your case has been mishandled.

While social workers don't make decisions for you or steer you toward making a particular choice, they can and do provide you with all the information you want and need, or they can put you in touch with the appropriate office or individual.

Most hospitals, including Cleveland Clinic, have a patient-care center or office of patient support services, where staff members review your medical concerns and talk with doctors, nurses, social workers, or others to resolve your questions and make sure that you are receiving timely and appropriate care.

Most hospitals also have an ombudsman available. An ombudsman is a member of the hospital staff (often trained as a social worker or a nurse) who is available to help you to deal with hospital-based problems or complaints. For example, if you receive a bill for a service you didn't receive, or if you feel that your medical or nursing team is not responding to your concerns or issues appropriately, you can speak confidentially with the ombudsman. After gathering the necessary information, the ombudsman can advise you about the steps to take and sometimes will simply represent your interests to resolve the problem.

There are also public or government organizations that provide advocacy for patient safety.

- If you have a complaint about your doctor, the American Medical Association will investigate and, if appropriate, take action. Contact your state medical board for more information; www.ama-assn.org/ama/pub/category/2645.html provides state links.

- If your concern is about your hospital, surgical center or laboratory, contact the Joint Commission on Accreditation of Health Care Organizations (http://jcwebnoc.jcaho.org/QMS Internet/IncidentEntry.aspx).

- The U.S. government operates the Agency for Healthcare Research and Quality (www.ahrq.gov), which investigates cases involving patient safety.

- The U.S. government's Food and Drug Administration investigates problems with medications or medical devices through its MedWatch reporting system; https://www.access data.fda.gov/scripts/medwatch/medwatch-online.htm provides an online reporting form.

- Some of these agencies may require that you document your complaint or problem with copies of your medical records and supporting information. Federal law gives you the right to obtain a copy of your medical records. For a list of state guides to obtaining medical records, go to http://medicalrecordrights.georgetown.edu/records.html at the website of Georgetown University's Health Policy Institute.

- The federal government's Agency for Healthcare Research and Quality (www.ahrq.gov) and the National Institute of Health's Library of Medicine (www.nlm.nih.gov/medlineplus/patient safety.html) both offer many additional sources of information about patient safety and advocacy. ◆

BLADDER CANCER: SOME CLINICAL TRIALS

Social workers have detailed information on clinical trials and can put you in touch with reputable programs for which you might be eligible. Some of the health-care institutions conducting clinical trials in bladder cancer are:

- Cleveland Clinic Taussig Cancer Institute, www.clevelandclinic.org/cancer
- Memorial Sloan-Kettering Cancer Center, New York, New York, http://mskcc.org
- M.D. Anderson Cancer Center, Houston, Texas (University of Texas), http://mdanderson.org
- University of Michigan Comprehensive Cancer Center, Ann Arbor, Michigan, http://www.cancer.med.umich.edu
- Columbia University Medical Center, New York, New York, www.cumc.columbia.edu
- University of California, San Francisco, San Francisco, California, http://medschool.ucsf.edu/research
- Dana-Farber/Harvard Cancer Institute, Boston, Massachusetts, www.dfhcc.harvard.edu

Chapter 9

The Future

The future of bladder-cancer diagnosis and management is in the hands of patients and the medical profession.

Perhaps the biggest impediment to progress is the small proportion of patients who enter clinical trials. There are many reasons for this – doctors often are too busy to keep up to date with the available trials, and sometimes doctors just don't have connections that allow them to participate directly in clinical trials and they are reluctant to lose contact with their patients. Sometimes patients are fearful or just don't wish to make the commitment. The problem is that progress really only comes through clinical investigation, and at present not even 10 percent of eligible patients participate in the available studies.

Most promising for the future is the development of some of the novel targeted therapies – those that have been developed based upon our understanding of the biology of cancer, particularly the biochemistry and genetics of cancer. As mentioned previously, agents that are targeted on the inhibition of genes that control cancer growth (such as the epidermal growth factor receptor) and enzymes responsible for angiogenesis and cancer growth (such as the tyrosine kinase inhibitors) are perhaps the most promising current strategies.

We know that immunological stimulation, such as that offered by BCG for superficial bladder cancer, has been helpful in causing shrinkage of bladder cancer. There are a number of proteins that have been identified in the bladder that might constitute targets for immunological therapy, and clinical trials testing some of these new reagents are in progress.

In addition, several classes of novel anti-cancer compounds within the category of cytotoxic chemotherapy have recently been identified and are currently in phase I and phase II testing, trying to identify the safe dosage and likely anti-cancer effects against bladder cancer.

Another important area in the development of future strategies of cancer care will be in the area of molecular diagnostics. This involves the development of pathology tests that can identify specific genes or molecules within cancer cells that indicate prognosis or potential response to specific therapies.

For example, preliminary studies suggested that the P53 gene, a gene that suppresses cancer growth, can sometimes be mutated (or altered) in cancer of the bladder. Studies at the University of Southern California suggested that mutation of the P53 gene can be identified by a pathological test, that cancers with such mutations have a worse prognosis, and paradoxically that cancers with some of these mutations can actually have a better response to chemotherapy than those without the mutations. This set of observations was the subject of a large randomized trial that studied P53 mutations and response to chemotherapy in bladder cancer. That trial recently closed. The publication of these results may be important in shaping design strategies for future bladder-cancer trials.

What is very apparent is that our understanding of the drivers of cancer has become much clearer with our improved knowledge of the human genome (the components of the genes within the human body). As we design better drugs that are focused on the mechanisms of cancer growth, clinical trials will offer a greater potential for cure. However, this potential will also require our community, including patients, their families, and their doctors, to support the available trials, leading to a time when advanced bladder cancer is no longer such a threat. ◆

Appendix A

WHAT IS CANCER?

Cancer is not one disease; it is many diseases affecting parts of the human body. All cancers have one thing in common: Something has gone wrong in the way some of the body's cells normally grow, divide, and die.

In a healthy body, normal cells divide as new cells are needed (*mitosis*) and self-destruct when the cells become old or damaged (*apoptosis*).

However sometimes exposure to chemicals (for example, cigarette smoke), radiation, sunlight, or even rare types of virus infections, as well as heredity, can damage our DNA, those building blocks of our bodies that store our genetic material (genes).

When DNA is damaged, the genes that control cell growth may malfunction. For example, cells that normally act as "stoplights" during cell growth and division may break down. Sometimes the damage leads to the development of *oncogenes,* which stimulate uncontrolled cell growth. Sometimes the DNA damage leads to the absence of genes called *suppressor* genes, which normally function by preventing abnormal cells from growing into tumors.

When DNA is damaged and uncontrolled growth occurs, cancer cells invade the body. Sometimes the cancer cells cluster together to form a tumor. Tumors are "solid" cancers that affect the body's organs, such as the lungs, breast, bowel, prostate, or bladder. Other cancer cells don't form tumors and are "liquid," circulating in the bloodstream to cause cancers of the lymphatic and blood systems.

Cancers may remain clustered in a tumor or a specific area of the body, or they may invade surrounding or distant parts of the body.

In order to grow, tumors must build a system of blood vessels by a process called *angiogenesis.* Sometimes this process is interrupted by a physical, pharmaceutical, or chemical cause, and the tumor remains dormant.

Other times, the cancer cells or tumor do grow and may even invade other parts of the body. Sometimes cancer cells from an established tumor spread to surrounding tissue (invasion) or are transported through the bloodstream to other areas of the body (*metastasis*). For example, bladder-cancer cells may metastasize to the liver and tumors may appear there, although the tumors will still bei "bladder-cancer" cells even though they are physically present in the liver.

Different types of cancer behave differently. Even within a particular cancer type, such as bladder cancer, different forms of the disease have different characteristics and respond differently to treatment.

Appendix B

WEBSITES AND RESOURCES

While every effort has been made to suggest websites that are up-to-date, accurate, and professional, do check them out yourself to determine your level of confidence in the information provided. As recommended elsewhere in this book, please discuss any websites with your doctor before relying on the information provided on the website.

Evaluating Websites

The National Library of Medicine funds www.eaccesshealth.org/training/issues.html, a website that discusses how to determine whether you should trust medical information on a website. It includes a section on sites that are *not* recommended and links to services such as Quackwatch.

Cancer Index also provides a short evaluation form (at www.cancerindex.org/clinks18.htm) to help you determine whether websites are trustworthy and up-to-date.

Advanced Directives

FindLaw
http://estate.findlaw.com/estate-planning/living-wills.html
Provides information on living wills.

National Hospice and Palliative Care Organization
www.nhpco.org
1-800-658-8898
Provides links to state-by-state advanced directives, hospice programs, and Caring Connections, a comprehensive section on end-of-life issues.

Ohio Hospice and Palliative Care Organization

http://ohpco.org

1-800-776-9513

Offers links to hospices by city/area, with resources for hospice professionals as well as for families and hospice patients.

General Sites

The sites in this section include information about cancer. Many of these sites offer specific links to or information about bladder cancer, and some include extensive information not only on cancer, but on such subjects as support groups, grief, nutrition, oncology drugs, and clinical trials as well. Please discuss these sites and information you obtain from them with your doctor.

American Cancer Society

www.cancer.org

1-800-227-2345 or 1-800-ACS-2345

Includes a forum/message board, the Cancer Survivors Network, where you can ask questions, share information and resources, and talk with others dealing with cancer.

American Medical Association

www.ama-assn.org

1-800-621-8335

Includes a DoctorFinder and information on medical ethics.

American Society of Clinical Oncology

www.asco.org

A professional medical website that includes a section titled *PLWC, People Living With Cancer* (www.plwc.org/portal/site/PLWC).

Bladder Cancer Web Café

http://blcwebcafe.org/default.aspi

Provides inspiring stories of bladder-cancer survivors as well as online forums, resources, and information on bladder cancer.

CancerCare
www.cancercare.org
1-800-813-4673 or 1-800-813-HOPE
A nonprofit organization offering free professional support, including online support groups, for those with cancer.

Cancer Help Online
www.cancerhelponline.org
Provides links to thousands of cancer resources.

Cancer Index
www.cancerindex.org
A list of online cancer resources maintained by volunteers; the specific index for bladder cancer maintained on this site can be found at www.cancerindex.org/clinks3d.htm.

Chemocare.com
www.chemocare.com
Packed with information on how to manage chemotherapy and side effects as well as how to bank sperm, what to expect from various chemotherapy regimens, and much more. This website is affiliated with the program established by cancer survivor and Olympic gold medalist Scott Hamilton, the Scott Hamilton CARES Initiative, which can be found at www.clevelandclinic.org/cancer/scottcares.

Hospice of the Western Reserve
www.hospicewr.org
1-800-707-8922
Provides resources for caregivers, patients, and professionals.

Medline Plus
www.nlm.nih.gov/medlineplus
Lists detailed resources on cancer from the National Institutes of Health; includes a link to help you find local resources in your area.

National Coalition for Cancer Survivorship
http://www.canceradvocacy.org
1-877-622-7937 or 1-877-NCCS-YES
Includes an audio section titled "The Cancer Survival Toolbox."

National Cancer Institute

www.cancer.gov

1-800-422-6237 or 1-800-4-CANCER

Extensive resources include downloadable brochures, newsletters, a drug information list, live online help, and help finding a doctor for a second opinion.

National Institutes of Health

www.nih.gov

1-301-496-4000

Comprehensive website with resources on a wide range of cancer topics, information on clinical trials, and hotlines.

National Women's Health Information Center

www.4women.gov

1-800-994-9662

Offers general health information for women and girls from the U.S. Department of Health and Human Services.

Office of Minority Health

www.omhrc.gov

1-800-444-6472

Provides resources and information for African Americans, Native Americans, Latinos, Asian Americans, Hawaiians/Pacific Islanders.

Ohio Hospice and Palliative Care Organization

http://ohpco.org

1-800-776-9513

Gives links to hospices by city/area, with resources for hospice professionals as well as for families and hospice patients.

The Wellness Community

www.thewellnesscommunity.org

1-888-793-9355 or 1-888-793-WELL

Offers extensive resources, information about clinical trials, online support groups, and webcasts.

Second Opinions

The National Cancer Institute
www.cancer.gov
1-800-422-6237 or 1-800-4-CANCER
Has a referral service to treatment centers it supports.

The American Board of Medical Specialties
www.abms.org
Lists certified doctors on its website. (Click on the section for consumers.)

Cleveland Clinic
www.clevelandclinic.org/quality/choose/second.htm
1-800-223-2273
Offers an article discussing when and how to get a second opinion.

National Cancer Institute
www.cancer.gov/cancertopics/wyntk/ bladder/page9
1-800-422-6237 or 1-800-4-CANCER
Includes an article on getting a second opinion when the diagnosis is specifically bladder cancer.

Clinical Trials

Besides **Cleveland Clinic,** www.clevelandclinic.org/cancer, and the links provided in Chapter 6, the following websites have information on clinical trials, whether to participate, how to find and evaluate programs, and what's new.

American Association for Cancer Research
www.aacr.org
Offers a cancer dictionary, information on clinical trials, and the latest research.

National Cancer Institute
www.cancer.gov
1-800-422-6237 or 1-800-4-CANCER

U.S. National Institutes of Health
and the **National Library of Medicine**
www.clinicaltrials.gov
Provide information on federally funded and privately funded
clinical trials, searchable by disease, sponsor, and recruitment status.

Coping with Cancer and Grief

American Cancer Society
www.cancer.org
1-800-227-2345 or 1-800-ACS-2345
Provides information on coping with cancer, from diagnosis and
treatment issues to managing everyday life; includes the Cancer
Survivors Network, videos, and personal stories about coping
with cancer.

Books for children about cancer
www.cancer.med.umich.edu/learn/pwtalking.htm
A reading list provided by the University of Michigan.

CancerCare
www.cancercare.org
1-800-813-4673
Features a "reading room" with articles for those with cancer, loved
ones, and caregivers; online support groups; and a "get help" section
with online support.

Caregivers Library
www.caregiverslibrary.org
Provides articles, lists, and resources on caregiving, end-of-life
issues, and emotional support.

Cleveland Clinic Taussig Cancer Institute
1-866-223-8100 (Cancer Answer Line)
http://cms.clevelandclinic.org/cancer/default.cfm?id=1&oTopID=1

Cleveland Clinic 4th Angel Program

www.clevelandclinic.org/cancer/scottcares/4thangel/about.asp
1-800-223-2273, ext. 52573

Offers a mentorship program for those with cancer and their care givers; part of the Scott Hamilton CARES Initiative at Cleveland Clinic.

Cleveland Clinic Social Work Department

www.clevelandclinic.org/socialwork

Crisis, Grief & Healing

http://webhealing.com

Features online discussion boards for those dealing with grief and healing, excerpts of books and columns on grief, particularly for men, by a national psychotherapist.

Garments for those with urinary pouches can be ordered through Intimate Moments apparel at www.intimatemomentsapparel.com. Offers intimate and sports apparel.

Links to many apparel companies can be found at the website for Wound Ostomy and Continence Nurses Society, www.wocn.org; 1-888-224-9626.

Gillette Cancer Connection

www.gillettecancerconnect.org

Has sections for men and for women on living with cancer; offers downloadable brochures, including *When Someone You Love Has Cancer: A Guide for Families.*

Growth House

http://growthhouse.org

An exceptional resource on end of life and death with dignity; offers an online bookstore with topical titles and Quiet Music, a restful online radio channel.

Look Good, Feel Better

http://lookgoodfeelbetter.org

Its practical guides on personal appearance for men, women, and teens with cancer are available at the website or through a mail order video. Look Good, Feel Better has local "in person" programs throughout the world; the website includes a local program locator and you also can call 1-800-395-5665 (1-800-395-LOOK) to find a program in your area.

Mayo Clinic

www.mayoclinic.com/health/cancer-treatment/SA00071

Addresses the sexual side effects of cancer for women.

Mayo Clinic

www.mayoclinic.com/health/cancer-treatment/SA00070

Addresses the sexual side effects of cancer for men.

National Cancer Institute

www.cancer.gov/cancertopics/coping

1-800-422-6237 or 1-800-4-CANCER

Addresses comprehensive topics such as side effects, emotional concerns, pain, nutrition, and end-of-life concerns; includes an article on talking with children and teens about cancer: http://www.cancer.gov/cancertopics/When-Someone-You-Love-Is-Treated/page6.

National Coalition for Cancer Survivorship

http://www.canceradvocacy.org

1-877-622-7937

Includes an audio section entitled "The Cancer Survival Toolbox."

National Family Caregivers Association

www.nfcacares.org

Has tips, guides, and articles for caregivers.

National Hospice and Palliative Care Organization

www.nhpco.org

1-800-658-8898

Has links to state-by-state advance directives and hospice programs, and features Caring Connections, a comprehensive section on end of life.

OncoLink

www.oncolink.com/coping/index.cfm

Provides comprehensive information about cancer for patients, caregivers, and loved ones; includes an online ask-the-expert section and a section for newly diagnosed patients.

Drug Assistance and Oncology Drugs

Federal Food and Drug Administration

www.fda.gov/cder/cancer/index.htm

Oncology drug research and evaluation website, including a list of approved oncology drugs.

Needy Meds

www.needymeds.com

Lists most major drugs and drug company programs. (Some applications are available at the website.)

RxAssist

www.rxassist.org

1-877-844-8442

Lists drugs and drug company programs, with chart comparing most drug-discount programs.

Partners for Prescription Assistance

https://www.pparx.org/Intro.php

1-888-477-2669 or 1-888-4PPA-NOW

An interactive website sponsored by the Pharmaceutical Research and Manufacturers of America (PhRMA, www.phrma.org); links to 475 public and private programs helping eligible patients obtain free or nearly free medications.

There are also programs sponsored by individual pharmaceutical companies or by consortiums of pharmaceutical companies. This is a sample listing of available programs:

LillyMedicareAnswers

www.LillyMedicareAnswers.com

1-877-795-4559 or 1-877-RX-LILLY

Sponsored by Eli Lilly and Company for patients needing medications not covered by Medicare Part D.

Pfizer Sharecard

www.pfizer.com

For those age 65 or older or other Medicare enrollees; prescriptions cost $15 for a 30-day supply with a Sharecard.

SaveWell

www.savewell.com

1-877-728-3935 or 1-877-SAVEWELL

Administered by Medical Mutual of Ohio; offers discounted prescriptions as well as discounted vision and dental care.

Together Rx Card

www.togetherrxaccess.com

1-800-444-4106

Open to seniors and others on Medicare; offers discounted prescriptions from seven major pharmaceutical companies.

Orange Card

www.orangecard.com

1-888-672-6436 or 1-888-ORANGE6

Offers assistance for seniors and those on Medicare through GlaxoSmithKline pharmaceuticals.

Government Agencies

Centers for Disease Control

www.cdc.gov/cancer

Provides cancer statistics and resources for cancer prevention and control.

Medicaid

www.cms.hhs.gov/home/medicaid.asp

Has comprehensive links to information about Medicaid health care Medicare, www.medicare.gov (1-800-MEDICARE).

Medicare Rights Center

http://www.medicarerights.org

Offers an independent source of health-care information counseling, including a hotline for Medicare questions and an enrollment program for those who need help with medical care costs.

Social Security Administration

www.ssa.gov

1-800-772-1213

Information on Medicare, the Medicare prescription drug plan, disability insurance, and SSI (Supplemental Security Income).

U.S. Department of Health and Human Services

http://www.dhhs.gov

1-877-696-6775

Provides resources on drugs, bioethics, clinical trials, coping and support, alternative medicine, and specific diseases.

Help with Insurance, Financial Assistance, or Employment

Association of Community Cancer Centers

www.accc-cancer.org

1-301-984-9496

Offers article: "Cancer Treatments Your Insurance Should Cover."

CancerBackUp

www.cancerbackup.org.uk/Resourcessupport/Practicalissues/
Workcancer/Goingbacktowork

Information, practical advice, and support for cancer patients and their families, with extensive information on issues connected with the return to work.

CancerCare
www.cancercare.org/get_help/assistance/index.php
1-800-813-4673
Includes a printable booklet, A Helping Hand, giving resources and tips for finding financial assistance.

Civil Rights Offices
http://public.findlaw.com/civil-rights/civil-rights-resources/state-civil-rights-offices.html
A list of state civil rights offices (for discrimination complaints).

Healthinsuranceinfo.net
www.healthinsuranceinfo.net
A nonprofit website on how to get and keep health insurance; includes guides to managing medical bills and state-by-state consumer health guides written by the Georgetown University Health Policy Institute.

National Association of Insurance Commissioners
http://www.naic.org
1-816-842-3600
Has information about state insurance offices and links to state departments of insurance.

National Coalition for Cancer Survivorship
http://www.canceradvocacy.org/resources/publications
1-301-650-8868
Includes the article "What Cancer Survivors Need to Know About Health Insurance."

Patient Advocate Foundation
www.patientadvocate.org
1-800-532-5274
A national nonprofit organization helping patients deal with insurance companies, manage debt crisis, and liaise with employers; online support.

State Health Insurance Assistance Programs

www.shiptalk.org

A counseling program with information about health-insurance assistance for Medicare recipients.

U.S. Department of Labor

www.dol.gov

1-866-487-2365 or 1-866-4-USA-DOL

Gives information on Family Leave Act, COBRA insurance, Americans with Disabilities Act, and the Rehabilitation Act.

Miscellaneous Resources

Air Charity Network

http://aircharitynetwork.org

Executive offices: 1-877-858-7788

To request assistance: 1-877-621-7177

Provides assistance to people in need of free air transportation to specialized health-care facilities.

Cancer Patient Travel

www.cancerpatienttravel.org

Travel/administrative office: 1-757-318-9174

Travel/patient phone: 1-800-296-1217

Lodging: 1-800-542-9730

Organizes charitable long-distance travel and lodging for cancer patients in need.

Hope Lodge

www.cancer.org/docroot/SHR/content/ SHR_2.1_x_Hope_Lodge.asp

Provided by the American Cancer Society; helps with housing for families who need to be away from home for cancer treatment.

Joe's House

www.joeshouse.org

1-877-563-7468

A nonprofit organization specializing in accommodations for traveling cancer patients.

Online Medical and Health Information

AARP
www.aarp.org/health/staying_healthy/prevention/a2003-03-17-wwwhealth.html
Offers an article on "Finding Health Information Online."

Health on the Net Foundation
www.hon.ch/HONcode/ HONcodc_check.html
Provides the "Code of Conduct for Medical and Health Websites."

The Medical Library Association
http://mlanet.org/resources/medspeak/topten.html
A list of its top 10 most useful medical websites.

National Library of Medicine
Funds the website www.eaccesshealth.org/training/issues.html.

Quackwatch
www.quackwatch.org
A nonprofit website.

Appendix C

USING MEDICAL INFORMATION FROM THE INTERNET

Make sure the websites you visit are reputable. Some doctors already have lists of reputable websites that they give to patients interested in researching their diagnosis or treatment. In all cases, discuss any information you find online or elsewhere with your doctor.

Some things to look for when surfing the web for medical information:

- **Accuracy:** Can you verify the information elsewhere? Are sources cited? Are the sources professional?

- **Authority:** Who is the author? What are the author's credentials?

- **Objectivity:** Are there indications that the site wants to sell you something? Does it appear to have an "agenda" of some sort?

- **Timeliness:** When was the website last updated? Is it current? Are articles dated?

- **Principles:** Does the website state that it does not take the place of a doctor/patient relationship? Does it disclose any conflict of interest? Is advertising clearly marked as such? Is the website source a nonprofit group, a government agency, or a professional health organization? Is there a clearly identified way of contacting the webmaster or professionals cited on the website? Does it ask for any personal information, and if so, how does it protect confidential information?

Use the information you find to help you prepare questions for your medical team, educate yourself about a particular disease, and find helpful resources for such issues as insurance questions, finding a doctor or medical facility, and researching clinical trials. Do not use the information you find to diagnose yourself or self-prescribe a treatment plan. Websites are resources meant to enhance, not replace, health-care professionals.

Discuss the websites you visit and information you find with your doctor, but don't debate it or challenge his expertise. If your doctor feels that you are trying to put him on the spot rather than discuss your concerns or ask questions about information that you don't understand, he may become defensive. For example, don't bring in 50 or 60 pages of research and expect your doctor to read them. If you find an article from a reputable site that you want to discuss with your doctor, bring the relevant citation only, along with confirmation of the author and website's authenticity.

It is an indication of the extent of the information available on the Internet and the desire by providers that their patients be informed that many hospitals and large medical practices make computers available for patients to use.

You deserve a physician who values an educated, empowered patient, yet you don't want to empower yourself to the point of being an antagonist. It's a delicate balancing act for both patients and doctors, because while the Internet can be an important tool in the doctor/patient relationship, it can also be a wedge in the communication process and can, if not used properly, hinder your getting the best information available about your disease, diagnosis, and treatment.

Here are some websites concerned with safe use of the Internet for medical research:

http://www.eaccesshealth.org/training/issues.html
A website funded by the National Library of Medicine.

http://mlanet.org/resources/medspeak/topten.html
The Medical Library Association's list of its top 10 medical websites.

www.quackwatch.org
Quackwatch, a nonprofit website.

www.aarp.org/health/staying_healthy/prevention/a2003-03-17-wwwhealth.html
"Finding Health Information Online," an article on the AARP website.

www.hon.ch/HONcode/HONcode_check.html
The Code of Conduct for Medical and Health Websites provided by Health on the Net Foundation.

Here are some websites that both physicians and patients might find useful:

www.medstory.com
A search engine for medical information.

www.merckhomeedition.com
Site of *The Merck Manual of Medical Information.*

www.medem.com
An interactive site founded by the AMA.

Appendix D

HOW TO TALK
TO YOUR DOCTOR

Throughout this book we've talked about the importance of communicating with your doctor and discussing your questions and concerns during your journey through bladder cancer.

It might not seem so simple to you. You've been referred to a new doctor, a urologist, who is recommending chemotherapy and surgery. You wonder whether she even knows your name, and sometimes you feel as if she's rushing you because she has to move on to the next appointment. Yet she holds your life in her hands.

You'd like to communicate. But how?

Preparing for your doctor visits, especially during the diagnostic phase when you may be seeing a new doctor or a new team of doctors, is a good first step on your part.

One way to prepare is to organize your medical information.

Buy a three-ring notebook with some dividers in it, lots of blank sheets of notebook paper, and a three-hole paper punch. Mark the dividers with categories such as Medication, Tests and Results, Office Visits, Questions, Contacts. You'll find more categories as time goes by.

Take the notebook with you to appointments and even treatments if you want. Keep track of doctors' names, when you had what test, and when you started and stopped a particular treatment. It's easy to tape business cards or appointment reminders into the notebook, too. You'll have everything in one place, and it will help not only you but sometimes your doctor to keep track of things.

Keep track of your questions in your notebook; leave space to jot down a short answer. Some people like to use tape recorders to record their doctors' answers to questions. (Ask your doctor whether she minds; most don't.) Others prefer to bring someone with them to act as "extra ears." In either case, transfer the information to your notebook.

Do ask your doctor to write down or spell unfamiliar medical terms for you. It really helps when you can look them up in a medical dictionary. (A good online dictionary is www.nlm.nih.gov/medlineplus /mplusdictionary.html.)

Ask your questions in simple terms. *What is wrong with me? What do I do if this treatment fails? What does that drug do? Do I need a follow-up visit?* If you put your question in simple terms, you're more likely to receive an answer that's also couched in simple terms.

Sometimes doctors are so stressed by the pressures of their own lives, whether business or professional, that they hurry or become impatient. It's only human, but if you don't understand something, ask the doctor to repeat her answer. If you feel intimidated, remember: This is your life, your cancer, and you need to get answers. You *deserve* to have answers. Politely ask for an explanation.

And do be truthful. If you have four beers every night, don't fudge and say two. Smoking three cigarettes a week is still smoking, and an herbal supplement that you take to help you sleep can interact with other drugs; be sure you mention these things.

Don't hesitate to call the doctor's office if you forget to ask something or have a problem. If you want to talk to the doctor, not a nurse, it's reasonable to be firm, leave your number, and ask to be called back. It's not reasonable to demand that the doctor come to the phone while you wait.

Whether you are a new patient building a relationship with a new doctor or you are seeing the same doctor you've been going to for years, communication takes respect and a willingness to be open and professional.

It's well worth it.

Bibliography

The following represents a partial list of resources employed in the creation of this book.

Print Resources

Droller, MJ (ed.). *American Cancer Society Atlas of Clinical Oncology: Urothelial Tumors.* BC Decker, Inc., Hamilton, London, 2004.

Grossman HB, Natale RB, Tangen CM, et al. SWOG 8710 (INT-0080) –"Randomized phase III trial of neoadjuvant methotrexate, vinblastine, doxorubicin, and cisplatin + cystectomy versus cystectomy alone in patients with locally advanced bladder cancer." *New England Journal of Medicine*, 2003, 349, 859-66.

Raghavan D and Huben R. "Management of bladder cancer." *Current Problems in Cancer*, 1995; XIX:1-64.

Raghavan D, Scher H, Leibel S, and Lange P. *Principles and Practice of Genitourinary Oncology.* J. B. Lippincott-Raven, Philadelphia, 1997.

Raghavan D and Bailey MJ. *Bladder Cancer – Fast Facts*, second edition, Health Press, London, 2005

Resnick M and Novick A. *Urology Secrets*. Philadelphia, Hanley & Belfus, Inc., third edition, 2002.

Stein JP, Lieskovsky G, Cote R, et al. "Radical cystectomy in the treatment of invasive bladder cancer: Long-term results in 1054 patients." *Journal of Clinical Oncology*, 2001, 19: 666-675.

Online Resources

American Cancer Society (http://www.cancer.org). Numerous articles including (but not limited to) "Managing Your Cancer Experience," "Support Programs and Services," "Learn About Cancer," "Clinical Trials," and "Treatment Decision Tools."

American Society of Clinical Oncology (http://www.plwc.org). "People Living with Cancer," "Guide to Living with Bladder Cancer," and other articles.

Cleveland Clinic (www.clevelandclinic.org). Materials provided at the website and other materials published by Cleveland Clinic, including the homepages for Bladder Cancer, Clinical Trials, the Glickman Urological and Kidney Institute, the Scott Hamilton CARES Initiative, the sociology department, and the Taussig Cancer Institute.

National Cancer Institute (http://www.cancer.gov). Numerous articles including (but not limited to) "Cancer Topics," "Clinical Trials and Insurance Coverage: A Resource Guide," "Bladder Cancer," "Coping with Cancer," and "Cancer Statistics."

National Institutes of Health (http://health.nih.gov). Numerous articles including (but not limited to) Bladder Cancer home page, "What You Need to Know About Bladder Cancer," "General Cancer Resources," and "Dictionary of Cancer Terms."

National Institutes of Health/National Library of Medicine, Clinical Trials home page (http://www.clinicaltrials.gov).

National Hospice and Palliative Care Organization (http://www.nhpco.org). Numerous articles including (but not limited to) "Learn About End of Life Care," "Advance Directives," and "Caring Connections."

Index

OTHER BOOKS FROM CLEVELAND CLINIC PRESS

Age Well! A Cleveland Clinic Guide

Arthritis: A Cleveland Clinic Guide

Autopsy – Learning from the Dead: A Cleveland Clinic Guide

Battling the Beast Within: Success in Living with Adversity
(about multiple sclerosis)

Breastless in the City: A Young Woman's Story of Love, Loss,
and Breast Cancer

Epilepsy – Information for You and Those Who Care About You:
A Cleveland Clinic Guide

Forever Home
(a chapter book for young readers)

Getting a Good Night's Sleep: A Cleveland Clinic Guide

The Granny-Nanny: A Guide for Parents and Grandparents
Who Share Child Care

Headaches: A Cleveland Clinic Handbook

Heart Attack: A Cleveland Clinic Guide

Heroes with a Thousand Faces: True Stories of People with Facial
Deformities and Their Quest for Acceptance

Lessons Learned: Stroke Recovery from a Caregiver's Perspective

My Grampy Can't Walk
   (a children's picture book about multiple sclerosis)

One Stroke, Two Survivors
   (the journey of a stroke victim and his wife)

Overcoming Infertility: A Cleveland Clinic Guide

Planting the Roses: A Cancer Survivor's Story
   (about esophageal cancer)

Prostate Cancer: A Cleveland Clinic Guide

Sober Celebrations: Lively Entertaining Without the Spirits
   (alcohol-free cooking)

Stop Smoking Now! The Rewarding Journey to a Smoke-Free Life

Tango: Lessons for Life
   (a dancing doctor's perspective on healing and life)

Thyroid Disorders: A Cleveland Clinic Guide

To Act As A Unit: The Story of the Cleveland Clinic
   (fourth edition)

Transplanting a Face: Notes on a Life in Medicine

Women's Health – Your Body, Your Hormones, Your Choices:
   A Cleveland Clinic Guide

Write for Life: Healing Body, Mind, and Spirit Through
   Journal Writing

You and Your Cardiologist: A Cleveland Clinic Guide

You CAN Eat That! Awesome Food for Kids with Diabetes

CLEVELAND CLINIC PRESS

Cleveland Clinic Press publishes nonfiction trade books for the medical, health, nutrition, cookbook, and children's markets. It is the mission of the Press to increase the health literacy of the American public and to dispel myths and misinformation about medicine, health care, and treatment. Our authors include leading authorities from Cleveland Clinic as well as a diverse list of experts drawn from medical and health institutions whose research and treatment breakthroughs have helped countless people.

Each Cleveland Clinic Guide provides the health-care consumer with practical and authoritative information. Every book is reviewed for accuracy and timeliness by Cleveland Clinic experts.

www.clevelandclinicpress.org

CLEVELAND CLINIC

Cleveland Clinic, located in Cleveland, Ohio, is a not-for-profit multispecialty academic medical center that integrates clinical and hospital care with research and education. Cleveland Clinic was founded in 1921 by four renowned physicians with a vision of providing outstanding patient care based upon the principles of cooperation, compassion, and innovation. *U.S. News & World Report* consistently names Cleveland Clinic as one of the nation's best hospitals in its annual "America's Best Hospitals" survey. Approximately 1,800 full-time salaried physicians at Cleveland Clinic and Cleveland Clinic Florida represent more than 120 medical specialties and subspecialties. In 2006, patients came for treatment from every state and 100 countries.

www.clevelandclinic.org